# Beginner's Guide to Indoor Rowing

By Amanda Painter Diver, PT, DPT

Copyright @ 2020 by Amanda Painter Diver.
All rights reserved. No part of this book may be reproduced, stored, or transmitted by any means—whether auditory, graphic, mechanical, or electronic—without written permission of both publisher and author, except in the case of brief excerpts used in critical articles and reviews. Unauthorized reproduction of any part of this work is illegal and is punishable by law.

# Disclaimer

The information in this book is meant to supplement, not replace, proper rowing training. Like any sport involving speed, equipment, balance, strength, motor control, and environmental factors, rowing poses some inherent risk. The authors and publisher advise readers to take full responsibility for their safety and know their limits. Before practicing the skills described in this book, be sure that your equipment is well maintained and do not take risks beyond your level of experience, aptitude, training, and comfort level.

This book is not intended as a substitute for medical advice, even though the writer is a Doctor of Physical Therapy. The reader should regularly consult a health care provider in matters relating to his/her health and particularly with respect to any symptoms that may require diagnosis or medical attention.

# Dedication

There are countless people who have helped me along this journey of becoming a Physical Therapist, entrepreneur, and author. Words don't even seem to do it justice, but I want to say a heart-felt thank you to you all.

First, thank you to my husband, Aaron. Without you in my corner, I wouldn't be able to follow my dreams and this book would not exist. You are constantly supporting, encouraging, and pushing me to be the best version of myself and I truly thank you.

Second, thank you to the rest of my family. It truly does take a village and I am so glad to have an amazing village. Mom, you inspire and encourage me to dream big, follow my dreams, and never give up. Dad, thank you for always supporting and encouraging me to follow my dreams and helping support my dreams. Seeing as you were the first Painter author, I am following in your footsteps. Brother, Aaron, thank you for always being supportive and a great big brother. Also, thanks for writing a book too, as it truly seems to be a Painter tradition now. Sandy, you are the best godmother anyone could have and I am so glad to have you as my "second" mom. You support, encourage, and inspire me to be an amazing person and push myself everyday. Charles, thank you for also being there to support me and for all your patience and encouragement. So thank you family for supporting me throughout the years. I would not have been able to do this without any of you. I hope that one day I can repay you all for everything you have done, which is more than I can describe in words.

Lastly, thanks to so many others who have been amazingly supportive in my venture to become an entrepreneur and follow my dreams. And to Jeremy Sutton for the endless help getting this book out there!

# About the Author

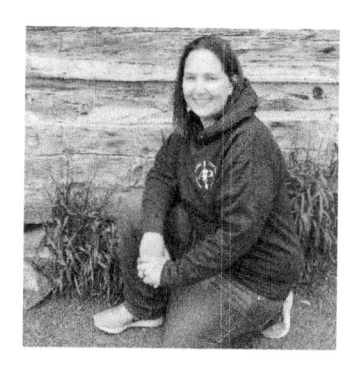

Dr. Amanda Painter Diver, PT, DPT is a Doctor of Physical Therapy living in Colorado with her husband and fur-kids. Amanda is the owner of *The Rowing Doc* and *Strong and Empowered Physio*.

Amanda has been rowing on and off the water since high school in 2001. She began her rowing career at Berkshire School in New England and continued by joining the crew team as a Division I rower at Santa Clara University. Shortly after graduation, she went on to get her Doctor of Physical Therapy degree at Samuel Merritt University. Her rowing experience combined with her passion to help people stay active and prevent injuries led her to start her own business helping both rowers on the water as well as the average gym-goer who uses the indoor rowing machine.

Amanda's career mission is to help people use the indoor rowing machine efficiently and without aches and pains. She wants everyone on a rowing machine to know what to do and how to row for their body type without being confused or overwhelmed. Amanda enjoys learning new things and helping people be the best versions of themselves. Her personal goal is to row across the Atlantic Ocean in December 2022.

## Table of Contents

*Introduction* ............................................................................... *ix*

*Chapter 1: WHY DO YOU ROW?* ........................................... *1*

*Chapter 2: SO WHAT IS GOOD FORM?* ................................. *7*

    Phases of the Rowing Stroke ........................................................ 9

*Chapter 3: WHAT ABOUT THE NUMBERS?* ........................ *13*

*Chapter 4: THE MACHINE DEMYSTIFIED* ............................ *23*

*Chapter 5: SET YOURSELF UP FOR SUCCESS* ..................... *31*

    The Damper Setting ................................................................... 33

    The Seat ...................................................................................... 34

    The Footplate ............................................................................. 36

    The Handle and Screen .............................................................. 37

*Chapter 6: PUTTING IT ALL TOGETHER* ............................. *41*

    The Stroke .................................................................................. 43

    Other Considerations During The Stroke .................................. 46

*Chapter 7: THE KEY IS IN THE WORKOUTS* ....................... *49*

*Chapter 8: I'M OUT OF BREATH…HELP* ............................. *55*

*Chapter 9: Gym Class Considerations* ............................... *63*

*Chapter 10: 4 WEEK WORKOUT PLAN* .............................. *67*

    Week 2 ........................................................................................ 70

    Week 3 ........................................................................................ 72

    Week 4 ........................................................................................ 74

*Chapter 11: FREQUENTLY ASKED QUESTIONS* .................. *77*

    What shoes should I wear? ........................................................ 79

    I walk duck-footed - what should I do? .................................... 81

    I get tailbone rashes - what do I do? ........................................ 82

I have a belly or am pregnant - what should I do?............................83

I get back pain - is this normal?......................................................84

I had back surgery - can I row?.......................................................84

I get blisters - should I wear gloves or use chalk to help keep the handle from slipping? ....................................................................85

I want to buy a rower – do you have any recommendations? ........86

*Want help or have questions? ..................................................92*

*Products ...................................................................................94*

   Rowing Consults ............................................................................94

   Forever Rowing .............................................................................94

   Rowing for PTs and Coaches .........................................................94

   Resilient Rower .............................................................................94

*References................................................................................98*

# Introduction

Why are you using the rowing machine?

- To stay fit and healthy?
- Keep the weight off or lose weight so you can travel and keep up with your friends?
- To avoid losing your independence and avoid joint replacements?
- Want your body to keep up with your mind as you get older?
- As a way to cross train from running?
- As a new form of exercise after an injury?
- As part of your workout routine in a gym class?

If your goal is to use the rowing machine for fitness, avoid getting hurt, and have some guidance along the way, then keep reading!

First off, thanks for showing interest in this book. It means you want to improve and you want to learn, and…you like the rowing machine! The indoor rowing machine is absolutely great at being a low-impact sport and useable by people of all ages, from kids to people in triple digits. Not only that, but it's great at improving whole body strength and cardiovascular endurance, and it sounds cool with its swoosh, swoosh with each pull of the handle. Even though the rowing machine is an amazing piece of equipment when used correctly, it can cause injuries if not used properly. If you decided to use the rowing machine because of an injury, it is a false notion that because the rowing machine is low impact, you can't get hurt. Have you ever met a rower, aka someone who does crew? Have you ever heard of them getting injured? It happens all the time. It happened to me as a rower. It happened to my husband on the indoor rowing machine. And it happens to tons of my clients. In fact, there was even a study done in 2012 that showed the most common injuries in rowers on and off the rowing machine are back, rib, and knee injuries.[1] This isn't meant to scare you. I am so happy that you enjoy rowing, and know that it is a great tool for workouts and to help prevent injuries, but please know that it can cause injuries if not done well. But that's what this book is for.

In the past 10 years, the indoor rowing machine has become more and more common in everyday life. They are in local gyms, CrossFit boxes, rowing team boathouses, and even living rooms. In the 1900's, rowing machines were most commonly found in boathouses so that people who rowed on the water and participated in the sport of Crew were able to row in the winter when the water was frozen over.[2] Rowing machines were and still are commonly used to learn the initial rowing mechanics and for time trials to get into a boat for a race. However, since these machines have become more common, there has been a drastic increase in the amount of people using the indoor rowing machine. While this sounds great, there are also less people being taught how to row well. I am hoping that this book is a stepping-stone to help people learn how to row well, so that less people get hurt from indoor rowing.

To put the rowing machine into perspective and how injuries can happen, think about Olympic Weightlifting, deadlifts, clean and jerks, or overhead squatting. These are all movements that are often done with a significant amount of weight. Since these movements require moving a lot of weight, people often focus on their form with less weight first, so that they won't get hurt as they lift more frequently or with more weight. This makes sense when we think of it that way, right? Now think about the treadmill, rowing machine, or stair master. These are pieces of exercise equipment that people usually just jump onto without any formal training. This makes sense for a treadmill and stair master, as these are movements we do every day. We climb stairs, which is like a stair master.

Many of us walk throughout the day, or maybe even run, and that's similar to the treadmill. But think about the rowing machine and how it isn't a natural movement, yet people use them at difficulty levels similar to those used by Olympic athletes who do crew. To jump on a rowing machine without any formal training will only limit your ability to accomplish your goals and could possibly result in increased risk of injury, which no one wants.[1]

Not only that, but a majority of people using the rowing machine these days aren't rowers on the water. Since they are more readily available and affordable, we see them in almost every gym. Rowing is more likely a means to an end for many people. They think of rowing as low impact, and as an alternative to running, walking, or the elliptical.[3] That is one of the amazing things about the rowing machine that has made it more popular. Get a great workout without the impact! Who wouldn't want to do that? I am one of those people. While I row on the water, I use the indoor rowing machine as a form of cardio exercise that is easy to fit into my life and workouts. It's a great full body workout, without any impact. Some people are runners, some people are rowers, some people are both. Personally, I hate running. I try to run every time I am near a beach, and when I trained for a triathlon, but it's not my thing. Every step is like torture. However since I grew up rowing on a crew team, the rowing machine comes easy to me and I like it way more than running, or the elliptical. Maybe you are like me, maybe you aren't, but whatever your reason is, that's what we want to focus on first and the rest will come.

People row for many reasons. Maybe you row for weight-loss; maybe you row so you won't be the last person on a hike and you want to increase your endurance; or maybe you want to stay active and strong so you don't need a hip or knee replacement. Whatever your reason for using the indoor rowing machine, I am glad you are here trying to learn more, and I truly hope you find and apply something useful in the following pages

BEGINNER'S GUIDE TO ROWING

# Chapter 1: WHY DO YOU ROW?

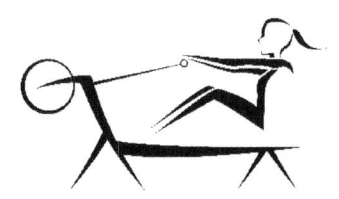

*Rowing is peaceful; it's my calm in the storm!*
— Amanda Painter Diver

BEGINNER'S GUIDE TO ROWING

## Chapter 1: Why do you row?

I know you are here to learn about the rowing machine. Either you are struggling to row for longer periods of time without being out of breath, or maybe you are brand new to rowing and want to stay injury-free and row well. Maybe you have been rowing for a couple of years, but now want to learn more. Perhaps you use rowing in your workout and want to be able to get a personal record (PR) on a benchmark or just want to stop hating the rowing machine. Either way, the first thing to figure out is... why do you want to row?

This might seem like a pretty basic question, but there are a lot of different answers. The more thought you put into figuring out the real reason that you want to row, the more you can define your goals and figure out how to achieve them. And I'm not talking about the simple, superficial answer, but rather the deeper reason. For example, you might say that you want to row longer periods of time so that you can lose weight. However, if I keep prodding and asking you questions, we might find that the reason you want to row and lose weight is so that you can have increased endurance. Keep asking yourself why.

But why do you want increased endurance? If we keep searching deeper and deeper, we might find that you workout three times a week with a trainer, but when you went on a trip with your friends, you were the slowest person and it frustrated you because some of the people were older and some of the people never workout. So why were you the slowest and out of breath when everyone else was having no problem? So then you blame being slow on being overweight and not working out enough. Granted, sometimes these things go hand in hand, but there are overweight people crushing their triathlon, cycling, running, and hiking goals every day.

BEGINNER'S GUIDE TO ROWING

The real reason may not be the first thing that pops into your brain when you say you want to improve your stamina. Yet, it definitely increases your motivation and desire to really succeed and push to improve your stamina beyond just wanting to lose weight. If weight loss is your goal, it's not likely that it's your first time trying to lose weight, and you probably know that motivation comes and goes in that regard. Finding motivation that goes deeper than the superficial gives you true motivation. It also gives you the real reason why you want to row, or workout, or whatever it is. Rowing longer periods with the end goal of not being the slowest person on your next trip is far more motivating than losing weight. Of course, if weight-loss happens along the way, fantastic, many of us won't object to that. I have been on my weight-loss journey since I was thirteen years old, on and off. The weight loss journey comes and goes, has ups and downs, that's why it's called a journey. But when I have a goal like hiking Machu Picchu, then I really push to improve, workout six days a week, and work to accomplish my goal. I didn't lose a ton of weight when I was eating amazing, working out a ton, and pushing myself towards my goal, however, I did feel stronger, more confident, more powerful, and happier in my body even though the scale didn't move. So while my goal was initially to lose weight, I found that even if the scale didn't move much, other areas of my life were improving. I felt better in my clothes. I felt strong lifting boxes of cat and dog food. I felt empowered to hike Machu Picchu. I needed to search deeper to find what I really wanted, which didn't really end up being about losing weight. It was about how I felt. I also wanted my blood pressure to improve, and it did, even though my dreaded BMI number never budged.

Perhaps you are in a gym like Orange Theory Fitness (OTF) or a CrossFit box (Box) where rowing is part of the workout. They do some benchmark rows throughout the year and maybe you want to get a PR. But why do you want to PR? Maybe it's to feel like a badass. But figure out why you really want to row better.

That's why this book starts here. Take some time to think about what your real deep reason is for rowing and why you want to row. By starting there, you are mentally setting yourself up for success. Rowing well and rowing longer isn't a quick fix, it takes time, so being mentally focused on your "why" will help you reach your goals.

Now that you know the "real" reason why you want to row, let's set a goal. Usually these two things go together, but not always.

In the example above, the person wanted to be able to row so that she wouldn't always be the last person on any adventure she went on with her friends. She believed that if she could row for 30 minutes, 5 times a week, she would have that accomplished. So she turned her desire of not wanting to be last into an endurance goal that she wanted to achieve.

So come up with what your goal is. If you don't set goals, you tend to not see or feel improvement. That being said, in order to see improvement, you also need to know where you are starting. So the last part of this chapter is to come up with a baseline. Where are you at now? Can you row for 500 meters? Maybe three minutes? How long can you row without needing to take a break? Write down where you are now so that you can see where you end up. Also pay attention to how it feels. Is your back aching? Are you having trouble because of your belly? Whatever it is, write it all down.

Later in this book, there is a four-week workout program that starts with a baseline row, which you can also use as a starting point. It is better to have tangible numbers rather than guessing, so keep the guessing to a minimum so you can see even the smallest of changes. Small changes add up. Think of it this way; if you were training for a half marathon, you're probably not going to run 13.1 miles on day one, or even on week one, maybe

## BEGINNER'S GUIDE TO ROWING

not even in the first month. Think of rowing in similar terms - don't expect to row 21,097 meters right away. It will take time to build up to that. Rowing often feels easier because it doesn't have impact, so we think we should be able to do more than we feel like we can, so just remember that rowing is hard on the body even if there is no impact and it still takes training to improve. You will get there, just give it some time, and some patience.

Action Step 1: Figure out the real reason why you want to row. Feel free to email me and share your "why". I would love to hear it! No joke, here is my email: amanda@rowingdoc.com

Action Step 2: As noted above, "success" is a journey and not a destination. Goals can be either short-term and regularly measured, or long-term as part of improving your quality of health and life. Now, create your rowing goals: distance, time, weight loss, etc. Be optimistic or realistic. Whatever it is, write it down.

My Why:


My Goal:

## Chapter 2: SO WHAT IS GOOD FORM?

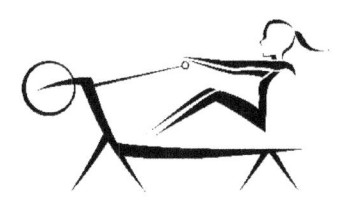

*Rushing is one of my biggest problems*
                                    - 3 seat

# BEGINNER'S GUIDE TO ROWING

## Chapter 2: So What Is Good Form?

Form. Form. Form. Everyone always says focus on form. Well...it's usually for a reason, even if it's repetitive and annoying. I get it, I just want to jump into a workout and get moving. But at a certain point, I realized that I would rather not get injured and the best way to help prevent injuries is by focusing on form.[1] Maybe it's because I have had three left ankle surgeries, which all started when I was about 14 years old, but I am all about form. Or perhaps it's because I am a Doctor of Physical Therapy. Who knows? Whether it is weightlifting or rowing, I would rather spend the time and focus on form, so I am less likely to get hurt from something I could've helped prevent.

Form is one of those things that takes time, and therefore gets annoying. It often means moving slower or not adding weight as quickly as others around you, but in the end, the person working on form is likely going to last longer without getting sidelined due to an injury. In fitness classes such as CrossFit, Rush Cycle, SoulCycle, Boot Camp, OTF, and just working out in general, people often get hurt.[4,5] Sometimes it's because they push themselves a little more than their bodies might be ready for and sometimes it's because they don't focus on form or just don't know the proper form. Whatever the reason is, and there are many, let's try and decrease your risk of getting an injury and not have rowing be the cause.

So now that we've established that I am a form guru, let me explain rowing form for you. I also highly recommend checking out my YouTube video on form, which is great for the visual learners. It can be found at: https://www.youtube.com/channel/UCb0crIZU9cLyGCxcJPYqcLA (or search Rowing Doc).

Phases of the Rowing Stroke

There are four different phases of the rowing stroke: **the catch, drive, finish,** and **recovery**.[6] Each part of the stroke has a purpose. As mentioned earlier, the rowing machine was designed for people who row on the water to be able to row off the water.[2] So, the different parts of the stroke relate to things that are happening with the oar and how it goes in and out of the water. You can see the different parts of the rowing stroke in Figure 2.1.

**The catch** is the part at the front of the stroke when you are all cramped up and compressed. Your knees and hips are bent, your ankles are at their maximum bend (dorsiflexed), your arms are straight, and you feel like your stomach has nowhere to go, or maybe that's just me since I have a belly. Either way, it's the part at the front. To relate this to the water, it's the part of the stroke where your oar has just been placed into the water and you are about to pull or push the oar through the water to move the boat.

Next is **the drive**. This is a really important part of the stroke. This is where lots of things can go "wrong". This is the part of the stroke where you are pushing really hard with your big leg muscles to move the oar through the water so you can get the boat to move. On the rowing machine, it's what affects the numbers on the screen to give you a split time (explained in Chapter 3) and tell you how much force you are applying. This is what makes you go faster. When I say faster, I mean if you are going 500 meters, it could take 3:30 or it could take 1:30. How hard you push with your legs and transmit the power through your legs to the machine affects these numbers. I will go over these numbers more in Chapter 3. But basically, it's the part of the stroke where you do all the work. You want to push with your legs, really hard.

At the end of the drive is **the finish**, because you finished the stroke. In the water, this is where the oar comes out of the water. It's the part where your knees are straight, hips more

## BEGINNER'S GUIDE TO ROWING

extended than before, core tight, and arms bent. You have finished moving the handle and are ready to start bringing the handle back to the front, **the catch**, position.

In order to get from the finish back to the catch, you have to go through **the recovery** phase of the rowing stroke. This part is called the recovery because it is when you get to recover and relax. It is also when you breathe and catch your breath from all the work you did in the drive phase of the stroke. However, this is also the part that many people aren't able to control, and it ends up being really quick, and therefore not a recovery period. This is the part that we will spend a lot of time focusing on. The others make sense. Start in a position, push really hard, and end in a position. But the recovery is where all the finesse comes in. Learn how to master the recovery, and you are well on your way to rowing for longer periods of time and not hating the rowing machine.

You might be wondering how the recovery period, when you aren't doing any work, can hold so much importance. Well, think of it this way. If you were to run a marathon, would you sprint the entire 26.2 miles, just as you would sprint a 100-meter dash? No! You would be so tired by the time you got to one mile that you would start walking the rest, or barely jogging. Rowing is the same concept and the part that controls that speed is the recovery. By going really quick on the recovery, you are essentially sprinting and by slowing down the recovery, you are learning to pace/jog. It's all in the recovery. Say it with me, "it's all in the recovery".

So master the recovery, learn to row longer and therefore increase your stamina on the rowing machine. TADA! Well, if it's that easy, why doesn't everyone go really slowly? Well, why don't you go slow? Because it's hard to master that slowness! Even in college on a Division 1 Crew team, most people have trouble slowing down the recovery. So, you are NOT alone. But, now that

BEGINNER'S GUIDE TO ROWING

you know the secret, let's go into the numbers and how you can tell if you are slowing down.

Figure 2.1:

Catch

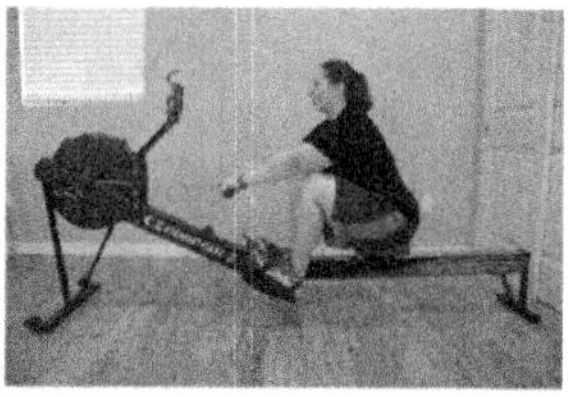

Drive

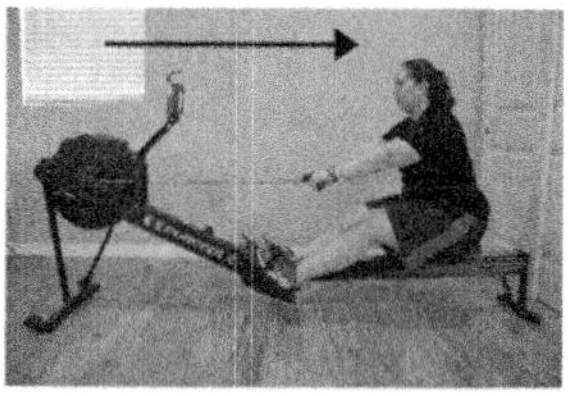

Finish

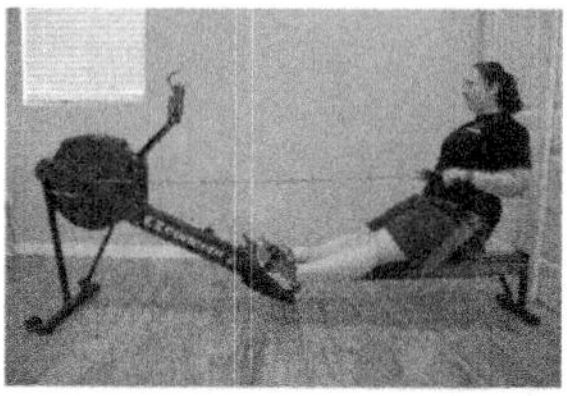

Recovery

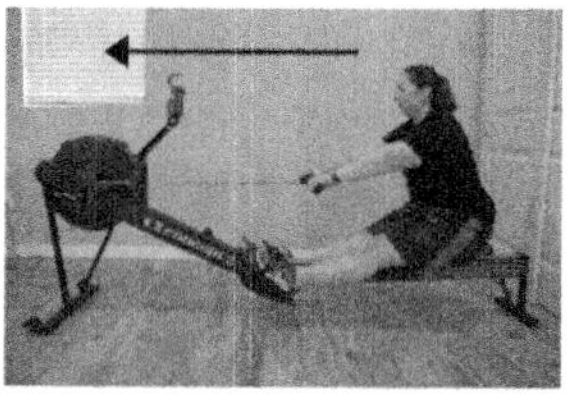

Action Step 1: Can you name the 4 components to the stroke?
　　　1.
　　　2.
　　　3.
　　　4.

# Chapter 3: WHAT ABOUT THE NUMBERS?

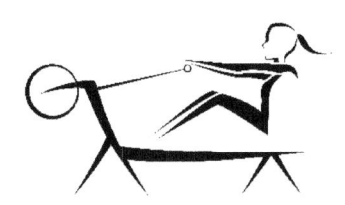

*I disliked numbers, and they didn't think much of me either.*
— R.J. Anderson, Ultraviolet

# BEGINNER'S GUIDE TO ROWING

## Chapter 3: What About The Numbers?

Numbers can be overwhelming. However, they can also give you a lot of data. First, don't be scared! This chapter is not going to go into depth about how the force curves should look, what pace is the best, or anything like that. My goal is to keep this simple and understandable. If you want more in-depth, there are plenty of YouTube videos that will explain it. Even the Concept2 website has information on what the force curve means.[7] I want you to understand the relevant numbers, what they mean, and how you affect them when you row, so you know how to change them if you want. This chapter will break the numbers down. I don't like to complicate things, but rather make it easy, so hopefully no one gets lost in this chapter. Now that you know how I like to keep things simple, let's get started.

Use Figure 3.2 and 3.3 at the end of this chapter as a reference point for this chapter. Figure 3.2 is from a Concept2 machine. If you are on a Concept2 machine, there are a few different options for screen display, so your screen may not look exactly like this. However, the numbers should be there, and if not, just change your screen display by pushing the "units" button repeatedly until it looks like this. If you aren't sure how to get here, you can press any button on the machine to turn it on, and then hit "just row". If you aren't on a Concept2 and you are using a WaterRower, Figure 3.3 is your reference point. For other indoor rowing machines like Lifestyle or any other, you can tell by the look of the numbers if it is what we are talking about, but it might be somewhere different on the screen. However, some machines leave out certain numbers, so if that is the case, feel free to reach out in the Facebook group (at the end of this book) and we are happy to help you decipher your machine.

Let's start with time (Figure 3.2: (a), Figure 3.3: (c)). This is the amount of time that you have rowed, counting upwards on this screen.[8] If you had chosen an amount of time to row instead of clicking "just row", this would count down, instead of up. But simply put, it's how long you have been rowing on the machine in that sitting. I haven't seen a rowing machine without this number, but I am sure someone will prove me wrong at some point. Most machines should tell you how long you have been rowing.

Next let's look at the Strokes Per Minute (SPM), or "S/M" on the machine, which means it is the amount of strokes you would take in one minute.[8] SPM is also often referred to as the stroke rate or stroke rating. See Figure 3.2: (c), Figure 3.3: (a). This is an important number and concept. This is usually a small number between 10-40. This is the number that really lets you know how fast or slow you are going. In a sprint portion of a race, this number is 30-40, but during other parts of rowing, it is usually lower, like 18-28.[9]

As I mentioned in Chapter 2, the recovery part of the stroke is when you go fast or slow, but more in terms of moving fast or slow back and forth on the machine. So if your seat is going really fast back and forth, you will have a higher SPM (like 30+). If your seat is moving really slow back and forth, you will have a lower SPM (like 18). The recovery is what really helps you control the SPM. It's important to understand that if you have an increased stroke rate, it doesn't mean you are working with greater intensity. The key to increasing intensity is knowing how to apply more power through the drive phase of the stroke. You want to get as much power as you can into each stroke (or drive), when you are pushing through your legs, not when you are moving the seat back to the front position (the recovery). Note that as your intensity increases (or how hard you are pushing increases), your pace per 500 meters will decrease, but your SPM does not need to change. So let's look at the pace I just mentioned.

The pace or split is essentially your workout intensity (Figure 3.2: (b), Figure 3.3: (b)).[8] This will change with every stroke, similar to the SPM. It is expressed as your pace per 500 meters. If we use running as an example, people say they run a 6-minute mile. Instead of using the mile, on the rowing machine we use 500 meters, so the pace could be two minutes (2:00) per 500 meters. Basically, it's how long it takes you to row 500 meters. The more intense your push is during the drive phase; this number will correlate with that. So if I push harder with my legs during the drive, my workout is more intense, and this number will decrease to show that you are going "faster". To put it another way, if you push harder with your legs, and are more powerful, then your pace improves. If you think of it in terms of running; if you are slower you may run a 13-minute mile, and if you are a fast runner, maybe your running is a 6-minute mile. These are two different paces. A 6-minute pace, and a 13-minute pace. So for rowing, if the number here decreased to say 1:50, you have a faster pace than if it reads 2:30 because it would take you 1:50 to go 500 meters instead of 2:30 to go 500 meters. The only thing that is changing is how much you are pushing through your legs on the drive. So *faster* relates more to how much force you are pushing through your legs, more than how fast you are moving your seat back and forth on the machine. People often confuse these two components and think faster must mean moving your seat faster. While this is the case sometimes, I think saying "*harder*" is a better way of telling people to row with more intensity because you are pushing *harder* with your legs.

Honestly, those two components we just talked about are the hardest ones, and yet the most important. If those two numbers make sense, you are well on your way to improving your endurance when rowing and not hating the rowing machine. The rest are a little more straightforward, like the first one we talked about in relation to time rowed.

Next is the average workout intensity, which is shown on a Concept2, but not on the main screen of a WaterRower (Figure 3.2: (e)).[8] This is measured as your pace per 500 meters like noted

17

above. However, instead of showing what your intensity is every stroke, this is the average for the 500 meters. If we think about how many strokes it would take to go 500 meters, it's roughly 50 strokes. A simple thought is that when rowing, if you row one stroke, you will go roughly 10 meters. I might have more intensity during some strokes and less for others, so this is the average, whereas Figure 3.2: (b), Figure 3.3: (b) is showing you what the intensity is for every stroke.[8]

The number of meters rowed, or total distance rowed is next (Figure 3.2: (d), Figure 3.3: (d)).[8] This is the total amount of meters you have rowed during the workout. If the screen turns off, this number, and all the others, will reset. So it's the distance you rowed during that workout period.

There are only two numbers left on the screen, and this is on a Concept2, not a WaterRower. The split time or pace (Figure 2: (f)) shows how your pace varied throughout the complete workout instead of the pace number that is just for that 500 meters you are rowing currently. The monitor will default to breaking a workout into fifths, so a split is 1/5 of the workout.[8] There are a few exceptions to this when you don't choose "just row" and you choose a preset distance like a 2000 meter row, or a marathon row for instance. For example, the splits for a 2000-meter row are 500 m each or ¼ of the entire row instead of 1/5. To be honest, unless you are really getting into following the numbers, this isn't too important. I only look at this when I am training for a competition, but on a daily basis, I don't look at it. I know this number is a little more complicated, but it's really not hugely important as a beginner. Honestly, I don't think I have looked at this split number since competing in college.

The last number is the projected finish (Figure 3.2: (g)). In this screen display, this is how many meters you would row in 30 minutes at the current intensity you are rowing at.[8] So basically, it's how far you will row if you row for 30 minutes without changing anything. This number will change based on your intensity (Figure 3.2: (b)). If you are doing a workout with a preset time, distance, or intervals, this number will be different and possibly even in different units. But if you are using the "just row" option, it will default to this.

      Hopefully this chapter didn't overwhelm you and you have a better understanding of what the numbers on the machine mean. If you can understand the numbers, figuring out how to improve becomes much easier. It's just like driving. You might know that if you push one pedal (gas), the car will go, and if you press the other (brake), the car will slow down. But if you are in a manual car and don't know anything about the gears, the car is going to be jerking up and down the street and it might not be a very pleasant experience. Once you figure out that the higher gear might be more useful at higher speeds, the car ride is now smoother. The indoor rowing machine is similar. Once you understand that you can control the numbers and how to control them through different parts of the rowing stroke, your rowing experience can improve. So now that you understand all the numbers, let's talk about the machine.

BEGINNER'S GUIDE TO ROWING

Figure 3.2 (Concept2):

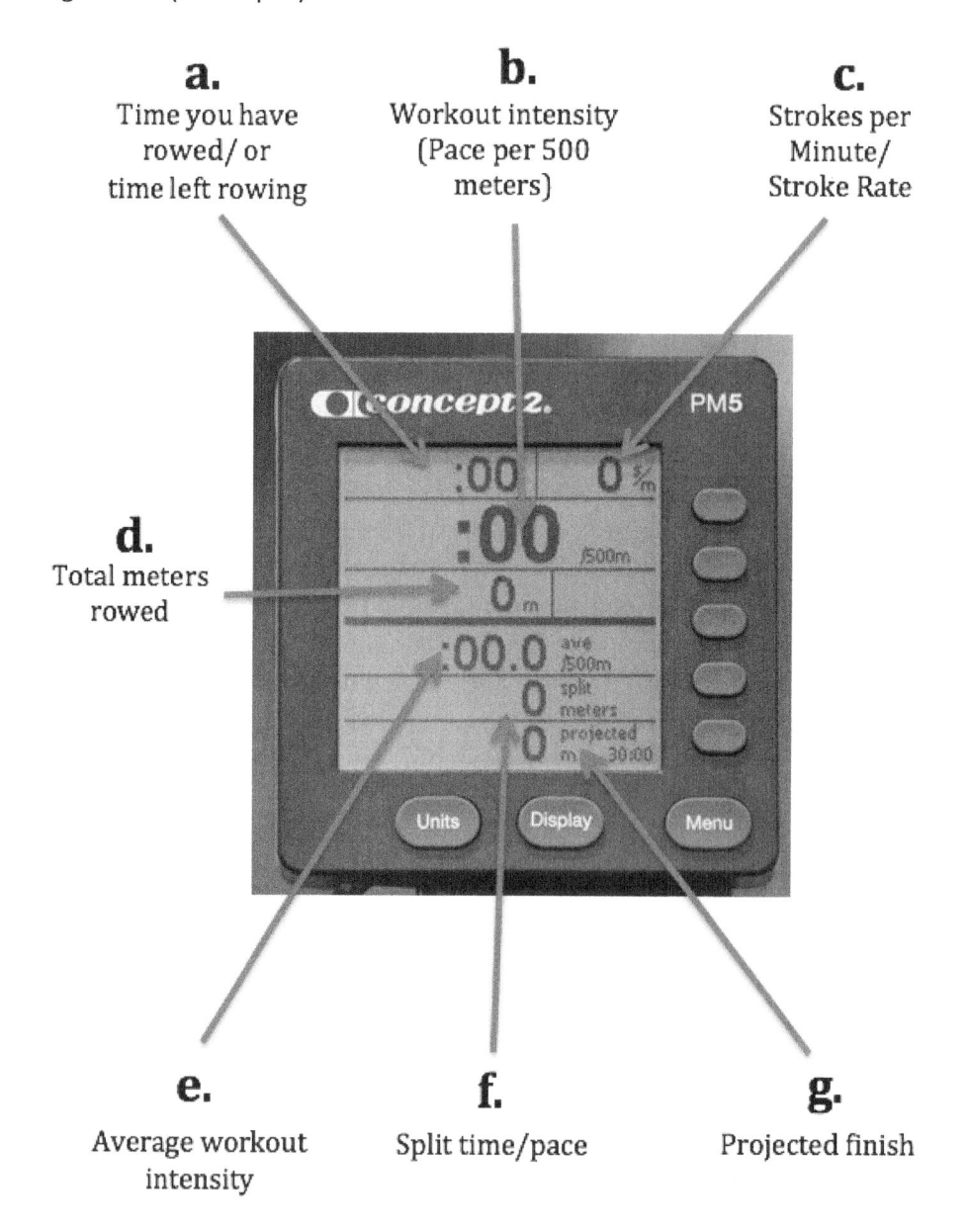

**a.**
Time you have rowed/ or time left rowing

**b.**
Workout intensity (Pace per 500 meters)

**c.**
Strokes per Minute/ Stroke Rate

**d.**
Total meters rowed

**e.**
Average workout intensity

**f.**
Split time/pace

**g.**
Projected finish

20

BEGINNER'S GUIDE TO ROWING

Figure 3.3 (WaterRower):

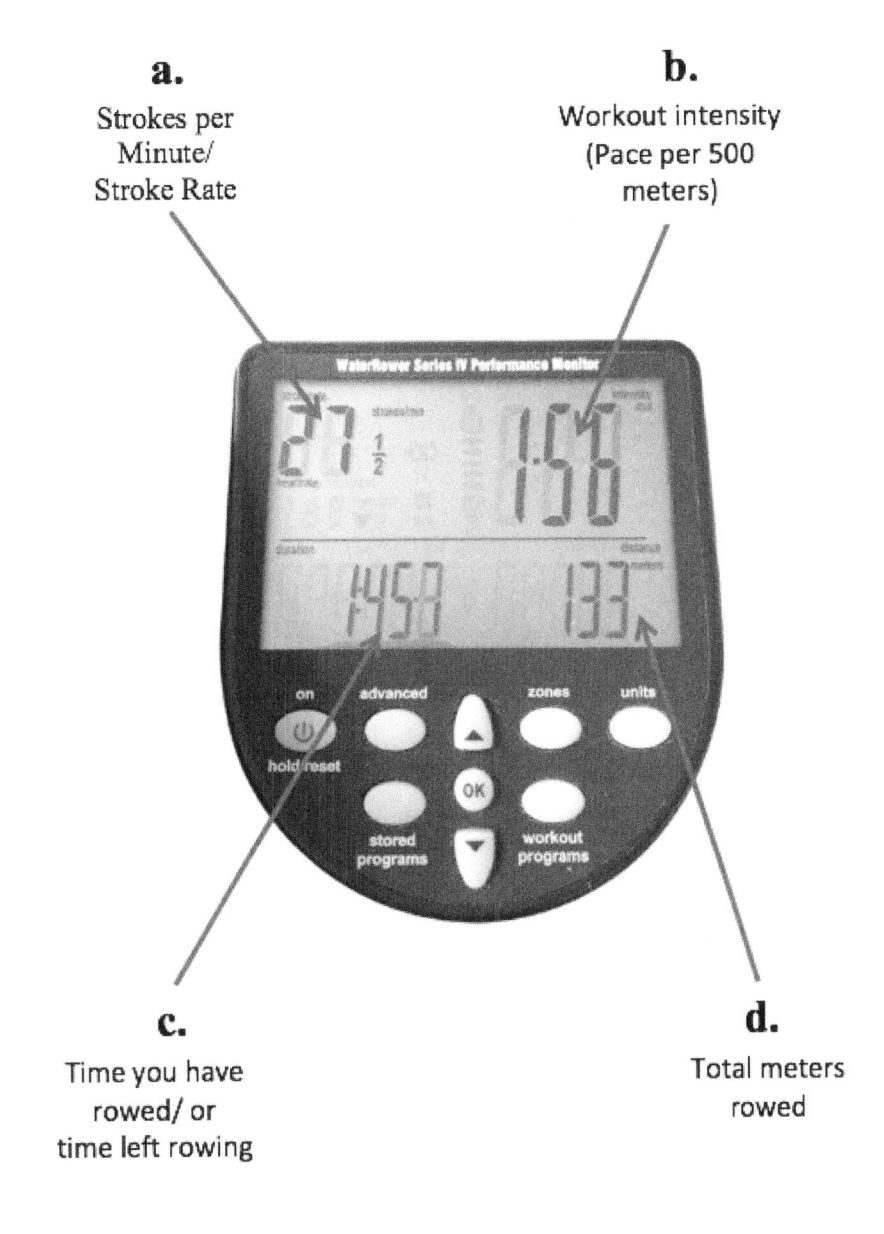

**a.**
Strokes per Minute/ Stroke Rate

**b.**
Workout intensity (Pace per 500 meters)

**c.**
Time you have rowed/ or time left rowing

**d.**
Total meters rowed

# BEGINNER'S GUIDE TO ROWING

# Chapter 4: THE MACHINE DEMYSTIFIED

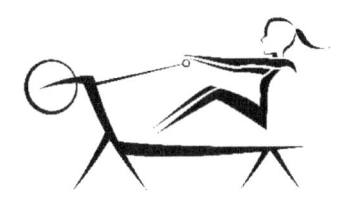

*Progress is made by the improvement of people, not the improvement of machines.*
— Adrian Tchaikovsky, Blood of the Mantis

BEGINNER'S GUIDE TO ROWING

## Chapter 4: The Machine Demystified

In this book I talk primarily about the Concept2, however I will point some things out in regard to the WaterRower as well. Each machine is slightly different in what it allows you to adjust, but for the most part, they are all very similar.

The key with rowing is that even though there is an "ideal" form, it's important to remember that we are not all the same. Shocking, I know. Every person has a slightly different body. I know that some people are different, but for the most part we are all the same in that we all breathe through a nose and mouth, we have muscles, skin, a heart, etc. Even though our core components are similar, we each have differences. I broke my ankle three times and had three left ankle surgeries, so my ankle is unique to me. Maybe you sit all day for a job and have never worked out. Or perhaps you were an elite level runner for twenty plus years and you are dealing with arthritis and trying not to have a knee replacement. Maybe you struggle with weight-loss and have a big tummy or thicker thighs. While some of these things are similar to other people, your body is unique to you. The rowing machine doesn't allow you to change a lot of things, but you can do your best to make the rowing machine work for you since you are unique, even if the machine isn't so unique.

I can't tell you how many times I was in CrossFit boxes, Rally Fitness, 24 Hour Fitness, OTF, or other gyms and watched people just hop on the rowing machine without changing anything. I don't know if these people didn't know they could change some things, or didn't care, or didn't know what to change to better help them. Regardless, this is why I am including this chapter. If no one ever teaches you, how can you know? Simple...you have to try it out or be taught. When we are infants, we try crawling and walking. When we are learning to do math, someone teaches us. It doesn't matter what way you learn; you learn it. So, let's start with what you can change on the indoor rowing machine.

See Figure 4.1 for a visual of the different parts of the rowing machine. While this image is from a Concept2, many of the components are present in other machines. All rowing machines should have a seat (f), so let's start there. It may not be comfortable, but it's what you sit on. Rowing is one of the few sports that has you sitting down. Now, most of you probably didn't think you could really sit "wrong" on the seat. While there is no "wrong" way, there is an optimal way to sit on the seat. I will explain what "optimal" is and why it matters in Chapter 5, but for this chapter, just know that there really isn't anything you can do to change the seat, except put some padding on. There are a bunch of companies making seat cushions now, but know that the thicker the cushion, the more it will change other parts of the rowing stroke. For instance, if you get a pad that adds 3 inches of padding, you will be sitting higher than was designed for the machine. So the angles for your hips, knees, and ankles will all change a little. It's not a bad thing, just something to consider. When it comes to the seat, I think of it as a necessary evil. It's similar to bike riding. The seat isn't comfortable, but as you ride more, your body gets used to it and adapts. The same goes for the rowing seat. The more you row, the more your body will get used to it.

The part of the rower that the seat is on is the track or slide (g). For the Concept2, it is a stainless-steel track. The biggest thing about the track is keeping it clean. Over time, it tends to build up with dust and leave some black marks on the track and not move as smoothly. You can take a tissue or cloth and just wipe down the track, no water or anything needed. You can even put a thin paper towel down, roll the seat over it back and forth and clean under the wheels that way. But the smoother you keep the track, the more pleasant the rowing.

The next part is the adjustable footplate (e) and straps. This is where you put your feet and strap your feet to the machine. Many people don't pay much attention to this; however, it can make a big difference if you change the setting to work best with your body. I will go more into how to set this up in Chapter 5, but a great place to start is with the strap around the widest part of your foot, which is often where the beginning lace part is on the shoe. There are reasons you might want to go above or below this, but it's a great starting point.

The handle (d) is the wooden or plastic thing that you hold onto and grab to get the rower to move and get the machine to register the activity you are doing. The biggest thing with the handle is to not over grip it, which we will touch on more in the next chapter.

The Concept2 and some other machines have a thing on the side called a flywheel with a damper setting (c).[10] There is something that moves up and down on the right side of the machine and it is numbered 0-10. The damper setting can get pretty complicated, but the basic point is that it changes how much air is going through the flywheel (a), which changes how it feels when you pull on the handle and row. I will cover this more later, but know that air resistance machines have this, and machines like the WaterRower don't because they are water based. The amount of water in the machine is what changes how it feels when you row. Some air and magnetic resistance machines also have a damper setting in a different spot, so keep your eye out for those.

Lastly is the screen (b). On the Concept2, you can move the screen back and forth so that it is in front of you and you can keep your head in a neutral position while rowing and still see all the data. On the WaterRower, the screen is a little more down, so you can't change it as much, and depending on which model you have, you might be able to move the screen more on some versus

BEGINNER'S GUIDE TO ROWING

others. But unfortunately, some of these machines make you look down for the numbers, which is not ideal for your neck position, so just keep that in mind. You might want to have it linked up to a program on your phone and set it up so you can see that in front of you at eye level.

    Those are the main components to the indoor rowing machine and how you can change some parts of the machine to help you row more efficiently, however we will go more in depth on how you can change the machine for you and your body in Chapter 5.

BEGINNER'S GUIDE TO ROWING

Figure 4.1:

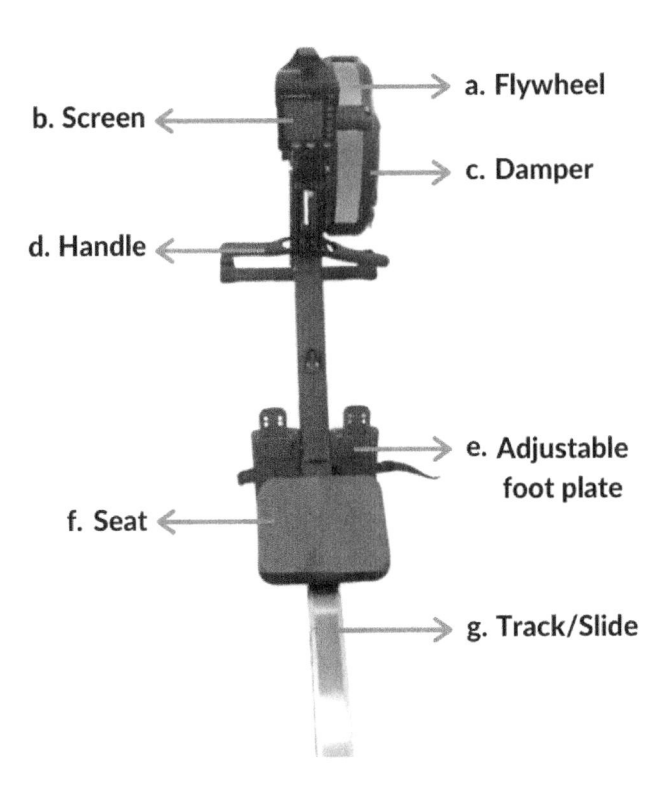

a. Flywheel
b. Screen
c. Damper
d. Handle
e. Adjustable foot plate
f. Seat
g. Track/Slide

# Chapter 5: SET YOUR SELF UP FOR SUCCESS

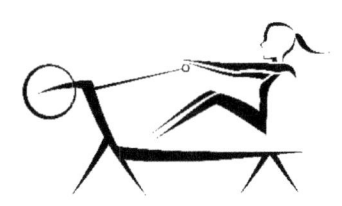

*I've failed over and over again in my life. And that is why I succeed.*

- Michael Jordan

## Chapter 5: Set Yourself Up For Success

I have mentioned it before, but I will mention it again. Not everybody is the same, and *every body* is different! That means that we won't all row the same. While there is the "optimal" rowing form and positioning, everyone has a different body with different circumstances and a different history. There are ways to make the rowing machine more comfortable and more optimal for you and your body and that is what we are going to cover in this chapter.

The Damper Setting

If you are on a Concept2, I recommend starting with the damper setting. Usually once you are strapped in and sitting down, it's hard to reach this setting, so doing it before you strap yourself in can be helpful. As I mentioned earlier, the damper setting can get complicated. So, I am going to try and keep this simple. The damper setting is basically how much air is coming into the flywheel. A higher damper setting lets more air into the flywheel and a lower number lets less air into it. The damper setting options range from 1-10. If you put it at a higher number, say 10, more air is coming in, and with a 1, less air is coming in. A great starting point is to put it at a 3-5. Most people who row on the water keep it somewhere in there.[10]

The way that I like to explain the damper setting is by comparing it to a bike. If you are going up a hill on a bike, you might have your bike gears at a really high setting and going up the hill feels impossible. So, then you lower the gears all the way and all of a sudden your pedals are moving super-fast and you feel like you are getting nowhere in regards to the hill. So, you go to a little higher of a gear (somewhere in the middle) and all of a sudden it feels comfortable and you feel like you are making progress. The resistance of the hill never changed, but how it felt to go up the hill changed based on the gear you were on. The damper setting is similar. Put it at a high number, 10, and it will feel really hard. Put it at a low number, 1, and it will feel really easy. Find a number somewhere in the middle, 3-6, and it feels comfortable. Some people like being at a higher number and some like being at a lower number. It's about finding what is comfortable for you and what you like. This can get a lot more complicated and you can start to look at the buffer setting, and I don't cover that in this book, but the Concept2 website has more information.[10] My goal is to keep this as a beginner's book, and from my experience, going into the buffer at this time would make it a lot more complicated.

## The Seat

Now let's start with the seat and sitting on it. You are probably thinking, "it's a seat, don't I just sit on it?" Well, you are half right. You do sit on it, but if you sit on the seat correctly, it will make everything else come a little easier in terms of positioning and posture.

Think about when you are sitting in a chair. You can sit in a slouched position, where your back is more rounded, and your pelvis is tilted forward (anterior pelvic tilt). In this sitting position, you're sitting more on your tailbone. Now if you sit up straight in a more upright position in the way that people say is "good posture", you will be in more of a neutral position with your pelvis and sitting on your sit-bones. Your sit bones are where you ideally want your weight to be going through when you sit because it means your body is stacked in a way that doesn't cause extra load on the spine.[11] But why does this matter in rowing? Great question! If you are sitting in a position that is more like a slouch, your hamstrings (the muscles in the back of your upper thigh) don't have as much tension on them. Additionally, it is actually harder for you to sit with a good neutral spine position. If you can't sit with a more upright spinal position, then you are compensating in other areas to get motion and putting extra stress on other areas to get you into certain positions in the rowing stroke. If you have a rounded back, then it will likely be harder for your upper back to get straight, which means when you get to the front catch position, your back will be more rounded throughout. This also means that when you get to the finish position at the end, you will likely compensate for a shorter length in stroke by leaning farther back. If you are creating all these compensations throughout the rowing movement, then you are more likely to have an injury either in the back, shoulder, ribs, hamstrings, or maybe even somewhere else, as your body is all connected.

     Hopefully this helps explain how just sitting on the seat can set you up for more or less success. Now there are some reasons that people often sit more in the slouched position. The most common reason is because of decreased hamstring flexibility. If you know this is the case for you, I recommend that you actually sit on your sit bones and make a change during the stroke to take some stress off the hamstrings and your nervous system. During the drive phase of the stroke, when you push with your legs, don't straighten your knees out all the way - stop with a tiny bend in the knees at the finish position. This is one of the adaptations you can make to help you stay injury-free longer. Another reason you might find yourself slouching and sitting on your tailbone is simply because you don't think about it and it is more comfortable because you can slouch more. Sitting up straight requires more core muscle use as well back muscle activation (posterior chain). If that is the case, with time, start working on your posture while rowing and just in your daily life, and this feeling of muscle fatigue in the back will gradually start to decrease. But if you can, try sitting on your sit bones on and off the rower to start making a habitual change. A third reason people often sit in a slouched position on their tailbone is because they lack flexibility or mobility in their mid-back (thoracic spine). If this is the case, I recommend doing your best to sit upright, and work on your thoracic mobility through other exercises, which can be found on my YouTube channel (link at end of book). Row in the range that is comfortable for you and adapt what you need to. That is the key to all of this.

Now that you know sitting on your sit bones is ideal, you might be wondering how the heck you get into that position. There are actually a couple of ways you can do this. One way is to sit on the seat, strap your feet in, and then lean forward as if you are going to touch your toes (Figure 5.1). This gives a little hamstring stretch and picks your buttocks up a little and gets you more onto your sit bones. Another way you can try is literally taking your hand and placing it on the bottom of your buttocks between the seat and your butt (Figure 5.2). Then lift your butt up and off the seat. Then repeat on the other side. This gets you more on your sit bones. Give it a shot.

## The Footplate

Next is the adjustable footplate. I mentioned in the previous chapter that a great place to start is with having the strap over the widest part of your foot, which is commonly over the beginning of your shoelaces. For many, this is perfect, however it isn't perfect for everyone. I usually recommend starting with this as a base and then after rowing for 5-6 times, try adjusting it if something doesn't quite feel right. Perhaps you get pinching in the front of your ankle at the catch position. That is a great reason to play with your foot position, among other reasons. The "optimal" positioning of your feet makes it so that your shinbones are perpendicular to the floor when you are at the catch position.[12] However, there are quite a few reasons people may not get into this "optimal" position, and that is okay. I personally haven't gotten into that position since rowing in high school, before having three left ankle surgeries, and I still rowed Division I in college. A majority of the population does not have the required ankle mobility to be able to get into that position, so changing your foot position can help you get close to that position because if you lower the foot plate, it requires less range of motion in your ankle to get you farther up the slide at the catch position. So, play with the position your ankle and the footplate are in so that you can experiment with what makes you and your body more comfortable.

The other thing about the footplate is that it varies between machines. On some machines the footplate is significantly lower in relation to the seat height. On some machines, like the WaterRower, the footplate is narrower. When looking at machines and when adjusting your positioning, all of these variables are important to consider. If you are a little thick-boned, or larger and wider, a narrow footplate might force your legs closer together, which will require different muscles to be used and might even put you in a position that your body might not like, possibly leading to injuries. There are footplate extenders you can get to attach to your machine, which will make the footplate less narrow, so that is something to consider. If the footplate is lower compared to the seat, it will change the angles at your ankles, knees, and hips when rowing, so try the machine and play around with what feels good for you when adjusting the foot plate.

## The Handle and Screen

There are a couple of things on the rowing machine that you can't really change. One is the handle and the other is the screen. On some machines, the screen can't be moved at all. On others, you might be able to position it more in front of your eyes so that you can keep your head forward instead of looking down, which might put more strain on your neck instead of being able to keep your neck in a neutral position while rowing, which is ideal. The "optimal" position is straight in front of your eyes, at eye level, so that you can keep your neck in a neutral position, without having to consistently look up or down while you are rowing.

BEGINNER'S GUIDE TO ROWING

As for the handle, the biggest thing is to not over grip the handle, and by that I mean, don't death-grip it. This can often lead to wrist, shoulder, or elbow aches and pains that aren't necessary and are easily avoided. If you do tend to over-grip, you can try having your thumb on the top of the handle instead of wrapped around the bottom. If you don't over-grip, then it is really personal preference on what is more comfortable for you.

However, the other part of the handle that you want to think about is where you place your hands on it. Try to keep your hands wider with your pinky over the side edge, as this will help keep your shoulders in a more neutral position as your hands will be about shoulder width apart and it will keep your hands from sliding inwards as you get sweaty during rowing. If you are a little wider, or have a belly, you also might want to look into the possibility of a handle replacement or add on, which can make the handle longer, which essentially makes it wider.

Now that you have some idea about the machine and how you can optimize the setup for you, remember to adjust the rower the next time you sit on it.


Rowing Checklist:
- Put the damper setting where you want it.
- Move the screen if you can so it's in front of your eyes.
- Adjust the footplate.
- Bring the handle so you can reach it.
- Set the monitor to the units that make sense to you.
- Get your buttocks in a good position - sit on your sit bones.
- Start rowing

BEGINNER'S GUIDE TO ROWING

Figure 5.1

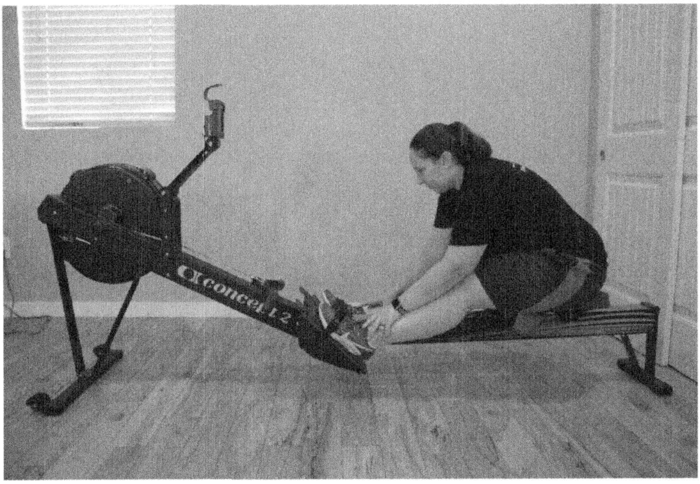

Figure 5.2

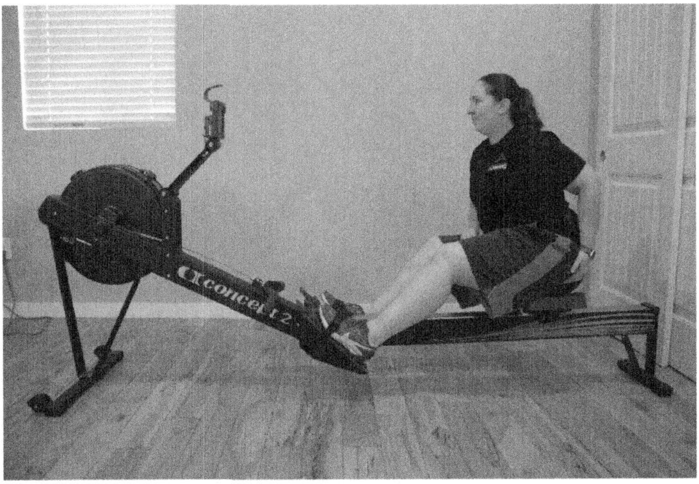

## Chapter 6: PUTTING IT ALL TOGETHER

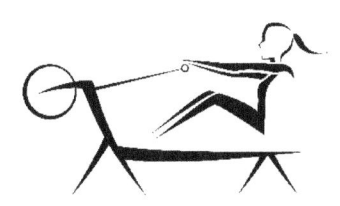

*Alone we can do so little; together we can do so much.*
                                          - Helen Keller

## Chapter 6: Putting it all together

Now that you know about the rowing machine, what you can change, and how to set yourself and the machine up for success, just hop on and start rowing. Just kidding. There is still more to learn about rowing. Rowing is a learned movement, meaning that it doesn't really come naturally to us. You know the main components to the rowing stroke. The catch. The drive. The finish. The recovery.[6] (Reference Figure 1 in Chapter 2 if you need a refresher.) Now, how do you actually get from one position to the next? Believe it or not, there is an order to your movement and there are three parts to the rowing stroke or movement.

## The Stroke

You might have heard it before, and you might not have, but here it is.... **Legs, Core, Arms** then reverse to **Arms, Core, Legs**. But what does that actually mean?

When you are at the catch position, with your buttocks in the right position, and you're holding onto the handle, the first thing that many people will say to do is "pull". However, this makes you want to pull with your arms first, when in reality, the first thing you want to do is actually push with your legs. 60% of the movement is done with the power of your legs.[13] What that means is that your leg muscles are the biggest muscles in your body, and they are doing most of the work. However, if you pull with your arms first, your weaker little arms are doing most of the work and it is more likely to cause injury to your upper body or back. So instead, push through your feet and use those big stronger leg muscles to really push yourself back by straightening your knees. The seat will slide backwards, and your legs will be straight. Then, once your legs are straight, you start to open up your hips, which is what I am calling "core". This action of opening up your hips creates a hinge like movement at your hips and involves moving from a slightly forward bent position to a slightly backwards position, and I say slightly because many people lean really far back, which is not ideal.

The hip hinge is an important part of the stroke that many people take out all together because it requires you to involve your core muscles. But the biggest thing here is that the core is what connects your arms and your legs in this movement, so if you skip this part, you are actually being less efficient on the rower and setting yourself up for injury because the core is less engaged and then you have something pushing at your legs and something pulling on your arms. It's like playing tug of war with your back and core. Imagine someone holding onto your legs and another person holding on to your hands. If you don't engage the core here, then you will flop around and while it may look funny, your body might not be so happy with you afterwards.

Knowing the importance of this part of the stroke, let's get into how to engage your core optimally and what this part of the movement actually looks like. I want you to think of a clock, with the ceiling being 12:00. Now depending on which way you are looking at yourself, your trunk movement is going to be moving back and forth between the 11 o'clock and 1 o'clock positions (roughly 30° forward and roughly 30° backwards).[1] So when you are at the catch position, your body is at 11:00, and then you push with your legs, straighten your knees, and then move your core/trunk to the finish position, which is at 1:00. So your trunk doesn't need to be almost parallel to the ground, which I see often, and is more likely to lead to low back injury.[1] Your trunk only moves a little, but that little bit makes a huge difference. Since this is a small movement, it is said that the core is involved in about 20% of the work for the rowing movement.[13]

The next part is arms. By this point, your legs have produced so much power, that the flywheel is already moving really quickly, and you don't need to produce much power with your arms to bring the handle in towards your body by bending

## BEGINNER'S GUIDE TO ROWING

your elbows. The arms produce roughly 20% of the power for the rowing stroke.[13] However, if you pull really hard with your arms at the beginning of the drive, then you are probably overusing them and making things harder for yourself and more likely to get an arm injury.[1] Now that your legs are straight, core is leaning back slightly to the 1:00 position, and your elbows are bent and the handle is in towards your body, you are finally in the finish position, so all of those three movements (legs, core, arms) made up the drive phase of the stroke.

Now to get back to the catch position, you go through the recovery phase. In chapter 2 we discussed the importance of this phase, however now you need to learn how to do it. In the drive phase that we just covered, you first push with your legs, then open your hips/core up, and then you bend your elbows in for the arms component. Well, for the recovery, we simply reverse it, so it would be arms, core, legs. When you are in the finish position, the next step is to quickly push your hands away from you and let the handle bring your arms in front of you by straightening your elbows. The recoil of the chain and the handle will help with this. Then once your elbows are straight, you close the angle at your hips, so your trunk goes from 1:00 back to the 11:00 position. Once your core/trunk is at that position, THEN you start bending your knees and do the leg portion of the stroke in reverse and this will return you to the catch position so that you are ready to begin the cycle all over again and row your next stroke. The big part to remember is that your arms should be straight before you start bending your knees.

Knowing the three main components to the stroke is a great starting point. I recommend spending some time focusing on this. At the beginning it will feel awkward, slow, and segmented. However, as you become more comfortable with the movement, it will start to get more smooth and natural feeling, with less pauses, and more continuous rowing without feeling jerky. So just keep practicing, and it will come with time. Although you now know the main components to the stroke, there are some other things to consider when rowing to help you stay injury free, which I will cover in the next section.

## Other Considerations During The Stroke

While knowing the legs-core-arms and arms-core-legs movement is key to working on your form, it is also important to look at your position at the catch, throughout the stroke, and at the finish. So I will cover some key points to consider while rowing.

Let's start with your positioning at the catch. One of the questions I get a lot is about posture and whether it matters. First, yes it does matter. Second, the catch is often where people struggle to maintain their posture. At the catch, it is common for people to lean forward and round their upper and mid back forward in a slouched position in an effort to reach farther forward. This is not an ideal position for your back or shoulders.[1] Instead, try sitting upright with a flatter back, but not so upright that you are over-extending at your back.

What happens when you lean forward at the catch and round your back is that you are putting extra strain on your back as soon as you start pushing with your legs. Sometimes this can lead to low back, upper back, or rib pains.[1] As for the shoulders, when you are in the catch position, with your back rounded, you lose the connection between your arms/handle and your body by having your arms really far out in front of you. The reason for this is because you have not engaged your back-shoulder muscles, which means you are relying more on your ligaments and arm muscles to initiate the rowing movement. So now that you know this positioning isn't ideal, what should you be doing? In the catch position, you want your back to be straight, but still hinged forward at the hips in that 11 o'clock position, core engaged and lats (back shoulder) engaged. In order to engage your lats, bring your shoulders back and down (like you are screwing your shoulder into your shoulder blade/back), which will pre-engage your shoulder muscles and this will help you stay more connected to the machine and help to engage all the muscles you want activated at that point in the movement as you begin the drive with your legs.

The next part that you want to spend some time on is the finish position. I mentioned it earlier, but here it is again. Try not to lean too far back in the finish position. Your trunk should be at the 1 o'clock position, with your core nice and strong and engaged. In this position you also want to look at your elbows, wrists, and shoulder positions.

One way you can start to look at this is actually by looking at the chain or band that is connected to the handle. When you are in the finish position, is the chain/band parallel to the ground, or is it going at a steep angle upwards? Your goal is to keep it as parallel to the ground as possible, which usually means pulling it lower than you think you need to, but this will vary depending on a person's height, so this will vary from person to person. Additionally, women usually want to pull a little lower, to the lower sternum area, to avoid running into their chests. The other way you can look at the position of your arms is by looking at each part of your arm. Are your shoulders really far out to the side, or are they down by the side of your body, or somewhere in between? If your shoulders are really far out to the side, then usually your elbows are far out to the side, and your wrists are often at an angle outwards (ulnar deviation). This causes extra stress on your shoulders, elbows, and wrists, and commonly results in an overuse injury.[1] If you keep your elbows a little more down towards the side of your body, when you pull your arms back, you can engage the back shoulder muscles (like you are pinching your shoulder blades together) and that helps protect your shoulder. With your shoulders in that position, your elbows are more down by your side, which keeps your wrists in more of a neutral position as well. As you are working on your form, it is good to sometimes look down at yourself in the finish position and see what position your wrists are in. Are the wrists bent up? Down? Sideways? These are all things that could contribute to a possible tendonitis and you might want to pay attention to this while you are starting out.[1]

The last part that we haven't really covered is in the drive phase of the stroke. When pushing through your feet, where do you push through? When you are at the catch, it is common to have your heels lifted up, which means as soon as you start pushing through your feet during the drive, you will be pushing with your toes. This is completely fine unless you are getting some lower leg symptoms, however, once you can get your heels down onto the foot plate, shift your weight so that you are pushing through your entire foot. A common error happens towards the finish, where you want to make sure your foot is still on the footplate. As some people get closer to the finish, they find they are only pushing through the heel, in which case the person is probably relying on the straps to keep them from flying off the machine. This often means that you are overusing your toes and shin muscles, which can also lead to an injury. If you are using the rowing machine as a way to cross train from having shin splints from running, this is something you want to look at and consider.[14]

Chapter Review Questions:

What are the three parts of the rowing stroke?

Does posture matter?

# Chapter 7: THE KEY IS IN THE WORKOUTS

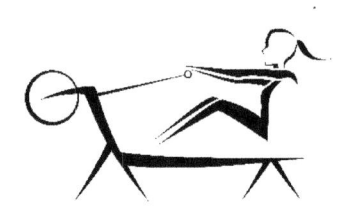

*All progress takes place outside the comfort zone.*
— Michael John Bobak

BEGINNER'S GUIDE TO ROWING

## Chapter 7: The key is in the workouts

Steady state. Platform. Intervals. HIIT. Tabata. Pyramid. These are some of the terms you might see floating around when you look up workouts for rowing. They each have their ups and downs and I am going to explain a little about what these workouts are and why they can be helpful. Remember though, my goal is to keep things simple for people. If you want to know more about any of these concepts, feel free to check out Dr. Google.

Let's start with Steady state. Steady state is a common term used in the rowing world to mean "continuous rowing at a consistent intensity and stroke rate for a set time or distance".[9] When doing this type of workout, the stroke rate is usually between 20-24 SPM, and it is usually performed at roughly 60-70% effort.[9] This basically means that you would work at 60-70% of your heart rate maximum, row for a long period (usually around 30+ minutes), at a consistent pace and stroke rate. Steady state rowing is great for cardiovascular endurance training, as well as for burning fat.[9] Longer periods of rowing are often associated with steady state rowing and are great at working the body's aerobic system.[15] Platform workouts are similar to steady state workouts, however the intensity level is higher at roughly 75-85% of effort. This is usually based on distance, so you would row a set distance, record the time, and try to beat your time on the next attempt.[9] An example of steady state and platform rowing would be rowing for 30 minutes, keeping your pace at 2:00 as consistently as you can, with an SPM of 22 as consistently as you can.

Intervals are similar to high intensity interval training (HIIT) and Tabata. Many people think that HIIT workouts need to be high impact, however this is not the case. HIIT is a "form of exercise in which short period of extremely demanding physical activity are alternated with less intense recovery periods"[17]. Simply put, it could be working really hard and getting your heart rate up with running in place, followed by some push-ups that demand strength, but allow your heart rate to decrease a bit. Tabata workouts are similar, however follow a more strict timeline and are often four minutes in duration for the activities.[18] It is usually 20 seconds of work, followed by 10 seconds of rest, repeated 8 times, for a total of 4 minutes. These workouts are also great at burning fat and getting your heart rate up.[15,16] In fact, there has been more research regarding Tabata workouts and fat loss and they have shown that you often burn calories for a longer period of time after working out when doing Tabata/interval style workouts.[19] In rowing terms, interval workouts are often "shorter periods of work at higher intensities followed by periods of 'rest'."[9] This can be based on time, distance, or amount of strokes taken in a period of time, however the goal is still often to get your heart rate up and is often done at 75-95% effort.[9]

The last common rowing workout is considered a pyramid workout. Pyramid workouts often "involve a gradual increase in work done followed by a gradual reduction in work done."[9] These workouts can be based on time, distance, or amount of strokes. An example of a pyramid workout is:

> 4:00 at SPM of 22
> 3:00 at SPM of 24
> 2:00 at SPM of 26
> 1:00 at SPM of 28
> 2:00 at SPM of 26
> 3:00 at SPM of 24
> 4:00 at SPM of 22

You could also stop in the middle at the 1:00 and that would be considered a half pyramid workout.[9]

A well-balanced program usually consists of a combination of these types of workouts. If you consistently do one over

## BEGINNER'S GUIDE TO ROWING

another, you will be putting more emphasis on different aspects of training your body. It is also important to note that there is a lot of debate on HIIT versus steady state rowing and weight loss, however that consensus seems to be that both result in decreased body weight and BMI, although interval workouts have been shown to increase weight loss even after the workout.[16,19,20] So if weight loss is your goal, there is actually mixed evidence. However adding a combination of different workouts to your routine is more likely to be beneficial if you are at a plateau.[21] This is why it is really important to know your goals and why you are rowing. If your goal is to increase endurance because you want to be able to last 8 hours on a mountain, then more steady state workouts might benefit you more than aiming strictly for weight loss and doing more interval training. Knowing your goals can really help direct you to the best workout for you. Usually programming has a mix of different types of workouts so that you have variety and are less likely to get bored, as well as to provide a different type of workout for different aspects of your body to help you reach your fitness goals.[19]

## Chapter 8: I'M OUT OF BREATH...HELP

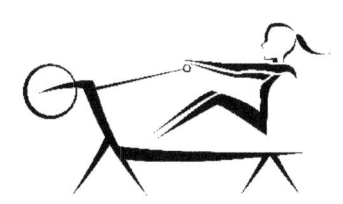

*If you want to conquer the anxiety of life, live in the moment, live in the breath.*
- Amit Ray, Om Chanting and Meditation

## Chapter 8: I'm out of breath...HELP

Being out of breath is a common occurrence with beginner rowers. However, just because you are out of breath doesn't mean that your cardiovascular endurance is bad. Instead, you need to understand why you are out of breath, and there are a few reasons that people often run out of breath when rowing. Figuring out which one of these, or how many of these, you are doing, or not doing, will help you pinpoint how to fix it and therefore how to row for longer periods and improve your stamina. Simply put, the reasons could be form related, speed control, breathing related, strength deficits, decreased cardiovascular endurance, and/or lack of training plans.

The first possibility is that you might need to work on your rowing form. I know, everyone always says to work on form, but that must mean that there is some truth to it. The thing about form is that it takes time to perfect. Therefore, people don't always take the time to learn it the "right" way. Some people never decide to work on the form, some people were never taught, some people were taught, but not well, some people were taught and are still working on it, some people try to learn the form later on, and others just simply don't care. Regardless of what category you fall into, even Olympic rowers are still working on their form, so there is always something that can be improved upon. I am by no means perfect, and still need to work on things. I think that when someone can admit that they aren't perfect and strives to always be better it makes them a better person and athlete.

If form can always be improved, then it's probably something you want to spend some time on. But you might be wondering how focusing on rowing form can help improve your stamina. This is a great question.

BEGINNER'S GUIDE TO ROWING

The most common reason that people are out of breath when rowing is because they can't really slow down when rowing. This also happens for a couple of reasons, but I believe that if you understand the numbers to the rowing machine, and how your rowing affects those numbers, you can start to slow down, which is why I cover the numbers on the machine so early on in this book in Chapter 3.

How you control the numbers on the screen is closely related to your rowing form and rowing speed. When you row, are you able to get the stroke rate below 20? Some of you might be saying, "What the heck is stroke rate?" in which case go back and re-read Chapter 3. Or maybe you're thinking, "Yah right, I row at 30 SPM." Getting an understanding of the numbers, what they mean, and how you can control them, can significantly improve one's stamina. The way that I like to explain the speed and trouble slowing down on the rower is by relating it to running, which we talked about a little bit in Chapter 3 in regards to the pacing. If you are going really fast with an SPM of 30, and you are doing that for 10+ minutes, that is essentially like trying to sprint for 10+ minutes. In running, if you are sprinting 100 meters, you are going to have a faster pace than if you are running a mile, in which case you will slow down a little because you know that you will be out of breath and start walking before you get close to the mile mark. Rowing is no different. Holding a 30 SPM speed for a long time is hard, and you should be out of breath or breathing heavier after 30 minutes at that pace. However, if you can learn to control the slide, and really take your time on the recovery, than you will be able to decrease your stroke rating (SPM) and last longer on the rowing machine without being out of breath. Some of this comes down to your form on the rower. Without good form, it's difficult to control the components of the rowing stroke and actually gain control of your stroke rating.[22]

A third reason that you might be struggling to breathe when rowing is because you are holding your breath or simply don't know when or how to breathe when rowing. This is commonly coupled with the second reason we talked about with going really fast, however not always. Have you ever been taught how to lift weights or in a yoga class taught how to breathe? Well, there are two ways you can breathe when rowing. Once is similar to what you might have learned with weightlifting or Pilates or yoga, where you breathe out when you are doing the part that requires exertion, and breathe in when you are doing the "easier" part. For instance, with a bicep curl, when you bring the weight up towards your chest and bend your elbow, you would breathe out. When you lower the weight back down to the floor and straighten your elbow, you breathe in. Then it repeats itself for the next bicep curl. In rowing, this strategy would be to breathe in when you are going forward on the recovery and breathe out when you are pushing with your legs in the drive phase. This works really well if you are going the perfect speed (SPM), but there are variations to this. For instance, if I am going 20 SPM, I might breathe out during the drive phase, and then breathe in, out, and in again during the recovery, and then out during the drive again. So this will look different for everyone and becomes a little harder to follow at higher stroke rates.

The other technique for breathing is to not really think about it, except remember to breathe, and don't hold your breath.[22] Back to the running analogy, when you run, you don't necessarily think about breathing. When you run faster, you breathe heavier, and when you slow down you "catch your breath" and breathe slower. So, in rowing, if you are at an SPM of 20, you would be breathing more slowly than if you are at an SPM of 30 where you would be breathing more heavily. This requires less thinking, but if you find that you have trouble breathing, maybe try the first method for a little bit and see how it works for you. For me, I row with this method, and when I do "power" strokes, I breathe with the first method. In case you are wondering what a "power" stroke is, it is when you keep the SPM the same, but instead of continuing at the same pace, you increase your pace and push really hard with your legs for a certain amount of strokes. A power 10, would be 10 strokes with more power. A power 20 is 20 strokes with more power. It is a way to refocus your energy while rowing when you find yourself slouching, losing focus, or falling behind in a race.

Whichever breathing technique you choose; everyone is different so there really is no right or wrong way. As long as you are remembering to breathe and don't hold your breath, your breathing while rowing will improve.

Another reason that people sometimes have trouble with rowing stamina and breathing is due to their decreased overall strength and cardiovascular endurance. You might be thinking, that's why I am rowing, to improve that. This actually comes down more to strength than cardiovascular endurance, unless you have an underlying medical condition that is contributing to a decrease in cardiovascular endurance. Your body has a bunch of fibers in the muscles and some are great for short term things like sprinting, while others are great for longer activities, like marathons. So you need to train the muscles that will help with longer activities in order to last longer. That comes down to a strength component. But you might be thinking, cardiovascular endurance is my heart…so why are you talking about muscles. Well, your heart is a muscle. It contracts and relaxes just like the muscles in your legs. We need to strengthen and train it to do what we want.

So that's the basics of how strength and cardiovascular endurance work together. It gets more complicated, but I am trying to keep things simple here. Strength is also important because sometimes people have trouble rowing for longer periods because certain aches and pains occur. This often happens due to poor form, or strength imbalances that cause increased strain on different areas and results in pains. So, if you work on getting muscles stronger, especially ones that aren't used as much in the rowing movement, you are more likely to help prevent injuries and imbalances from occurring. I can't guarantee you won't get hurt, as things do happen, but you can help decrease that likelihood.

Another common reason that you might get out of breath as it is related to strength is because you are overusing your arms. You might be saying, "That makes no sense!" But let me explain. Your legs are farther from your heart than your arms are. So when you use your arms more heavily, it actually puts an increased demand on your cardiovascular system then if you use your legs more. When people are rehabbing from an injury where they can't use their legs, we will often have people do arm exercises so that they can still work their cardiovascular system and get a workout, without using their legs. So if you are using your arms more than the 10-20% at the end of the drive phase in the rowing stroke, then you are likely putting increased demand on your cardiovascular system, and you will likely be out of breath more quickly.

In terms of cardiovascular endurance, maybe you have been sedentary for a few months. Maybe you were sick a couple of weeks ago and are struggling to get back to activity and this is the first thing you have done in a month. Whatever the reason is, you can build your endurance back up, just remember that it takes some time and patience. This leads us to another reason that you might be struggling. How you workout and try to improve your strength and cardiovascular endurance makes a huge difference. Just jumping on the rowing machine and rowing for 20 minutes every day, without a plan, can actually lead to stagnancy. In order to increase strength and cardiovascular endurance, we need to challenge our bodies and make them work differently so that they need to adapt and change. Having a plan can make a huge impact on your rowing stamina. Depending on what your goal with rowing is, that will impact what your rowing plan should be. Regardless, doing a mix of different strategies will be beneficial. Chapter 7 went more in-depth into this concept; however if you are looking to not be out of breath then the next chapter is great. Chapter 9 is a 4-week workout plan designed to help the beginner rower, or even someone who is experienced but hasn't really focused on everything mentioned in this book, row for 30+ minutes without being out of breath. I have a course that goes over everything in this book, and the workouts as well if you are interested or happen to learn more from visual cueing as opposed to reading, but this book has everything you need to be a successful rower.

    Now start rowing, remember to breathe, and congrats on taking the step to improving your rowing so you can reach all your rowing and non-rowing goals!

## Chapter 9: Gym Class Considerations

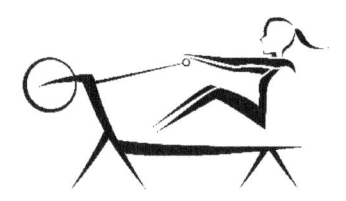

*Action is the foundational key to all success.*
                                  - Pablo Picasso

## Chapter 9: Gym Class Considerations

This is the chapter for those of you that do classes like OTF, CrossFit, or any other gym routine where rowing is part of the workout, but you get on and off the rower a lot.

In CrossFit, workouts are called the Workout of the Day (WOD). A WOD might be to do a 1000-meter row, followed by 50 squats, followed by 30 pull-ups, and the goal is to do it as quickly as possible. In this example, it would be similar to starting an OTF workout on the rower, going to the treadmill (tread), and then ending on the floor (strength training). In workouts that start on the rower and are quickly followed by a movement that is leg heavy like running, squats, or deadlifts, I usually recommend a certain strategy. A 1000-meter row is roughly 100 strokes, which is a lot. So when rowing, start out nice and strong, usually at a higher stroke rate of roughly 28-34 SPM, for roughly 20 strokes, or 200 meters. Then, settle down into a comfortable pace both in terms of your split and SPM. Towards the end, with roughly 100-150 meters left, instead of going all out and really pushing, I recommend actually backing off a little and using it as a cool down for those last 10ish strokes. That way your legs are all ready to go for your next leg-heavy movement and you won't lose a lot of time in your transition period. This is the same way I would approach the rowing section of a WOD if the rowing is in the middle of a workout or has a lot of rounds where you are going on and off of the rowing machine.

However, if the rowing is at the end of a WOD, don't ease up at the end. Instead, go a little gentler as a warm-up for the first 50-100 meters, then settle into a pace that is comfortable, and finish the last 200-250 meters with an all-out row, giving max effort so that you finish strong.

So if you think about your entire workout and do a little bit of planning for it, you can go in with a pretty solid strategy for being effective and getting the results you are looking for.

Now, if you are doing a benchmark workout like a 2k row, the strategy would be different, as you are really trying to beat a PR and do the best you can on the rower. In these instances, I recommend going in with a plan. If you go into a 2k with a strategy, like you approach your other workouts, you will feel more confident going into it and when you finish. I recently helped someone who said having a plan made the rowing way more manageable, and she felt more confident having a plan. So do some research and kill that benchmark row!

# Chapter 10: 4 WEEK WORKOUT PLAN

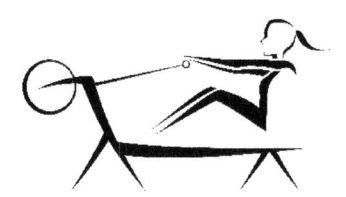

*The only bad workout is the one that didn't happen.*
— Anonymous

## Chapter 10: 4-week workout plan

This chapter is designed for beginners or people who are really looking to last longer on the rowing machine and not be out of breath after ten minutes. If you are a person who goes to a membership class such as OTF or CrossFit, this will work in conjunction with your classes, wherever you might be able to get on an indoor rowing machine. I have included how long the workouts should roughly take, and most of them are under 30 minutes, so you should be able to fit them into your routine.

**Week 1**

**Workout 1:**
Overview:
- Total Time: 15 min
- Rowing Time: 11 minutes, with 4 minutes of breaks
    - Row for 2 minutes at SPM of 24, comfortable effort, then rest 1 minute
    - Row for 2 minutes at SPM of 22, comfortable effort, then rest 1 minute
    - Row for 2 minutes at SPM of 20, comfortable effort, then rest 1 minute
    - Row for 2 minutes at SPM of 18, comfortable effort, then rest 1 minute
    - Then row 1 minute at SPM of 20, 1 minute at SPM of 22, and 1 minute at SPM of 24
- Afterwards, record:
    - How did it feel?

    - Total meters rowed?

**Workout 2:**
Overview:
- Total Time: 19 min
- Rowing Time: 15 minutes, with 2 - 2 minute breaks

BEGINNER'S GUIDE TO ROWING

- Row for 5 minutes, 3 times, with a varying stroke rate. Between each 5 minute piece, rest for 2 minutes.
  - For the first 2 minutes, row at 20 SPM
  - For the next 2 minutes, row at 18 SPM
  - For the last 1 minute, row at 20 SPM
  - Then rest and repeat
- Afterwards, record:
  - How did it feel?
  - Total meters rowed?

**Workout 3:**
Overview:
- Total Time: 22-25 min total
- Rowing Time: 10 minutes x 2, with 2-5 minutes of breaks between
  - Row for 10 minutes; focus on you and your form. How does it feel? Are you feeling achy anywhere? Are you out of breath? Record anything you feel after you row.
  - Take a 2-5 minute break, and row another 10 minutes.
- Afterwards, record:
  - How did it feel?
  - Total meters rowed?

Week 2

**Workout 1:**
Overview:
- Total Time: 16-36 min total depending on how many rounds you choose to do
- Rowing Time: 6 minutes x 2, 3, or 4. A short row or longer, it's up to you.
  - The goal is to focus on the stroke rate and the beginning parts of steady state rowing. That basically means trying to keep the stroke rate and the pace/split

as consistent as you can throughout the entire rowing piece.
    - Row for 6 minutes. Then take a 4-minute break. Repeat 1-3 more times, depending on how you are feeling. So row for 6 minutes, break for 4 minutes, row for 6 minutes, break for 4 minutes, and so forth. Between each piece, check in with yourself and write down how you are feeling.
    - Aim for a stroke rate between 18-22 throughout if you can.
- Afterwards, record:
    - How did it feel?
    - What distance did you row for each piece? Total?
    - What was the comfortable stroke rate that you settled into?

## Workout 2:

Overview:
- Total Time: 23 minutes
- Rowing Time: 10 minutes x 2, with a 3-minute break between.
    - Row for 10 minutes. To achieve the maximum benefit, it's important to properly pace each minute. Each minute will change a little, so you have to pay attention a little in this one.
    - Row with more force/power through your legs for 1 minute (1 minute hard), then row easy and gentle for 1 minute (1 minute easy). Then repeat this until 10 minutes is up. Then rest for 3 minutes and repeat once more.
    - So row 1 minute hard, 1 minute easy, 1 minute hard, 1 minute easy, until 10 minutes is up keep alternating.
    - Try to keep the stroke rate between 18-24 the entire time, so you are working on really pushing through the

BEGINNER'S GUIDE TO ROWING

legs in the drive, but also keeping the recovery nice and slow.
- Afterwards, record:
  - How did it feel?

  - Total meters rowed?

  - What stroke rate did you settle at?

**Workout 3:**
Overview:
- Total Time: Roughly under 25 minutes
- Rowing Time: Roughly 20 minutes
  - Row for 1000 meters, then rest for 1 minute
  - Row for 750 meters, then rest for 1 minute
  - Row for 500 meters, then rest for 1 minute
  - Row for 250 meters
  - Keep SPM below 24, even for the 250 meters, so really control the slide on the recovery.
- Afterwards, record:
  - How did it feel?

  - Total time it took?

  - What stroke rate did you settle at?

Week 3

**Workout 1:**
- Total Time: 15 minutes
- Rowing Time: 15 minutes
  - Row for 15 minutes
  - Focus on how it feels
  - Focus on different parts of the stroke

        - Aim for a feeling of smooth acceleration when pushing with the legs during the drive, and slow and relaxed on the recovery.
        - Try and make it all the way through without stopping.
- Afterwards, record:
    - Total meters rowed?
    - Average SPM you settled at?
    - How did it feel? Tired? Out of breath? Take a break?

**Workout 2:**
Overview:
- Total Time: Roughly 30 minutes
- Rowing Time: Roughly 22 minutes
    - Row 750 meters, 4 times, with a 2-minute break between each. So row 750 meters, rest 2-minutes, repeat 3 more times.
- Afterwards, record:
    - Average split/pace?
    - How long did it take?
    - How did it feel?

**Workout 3:**
Overview:
- Total Time: 30 minutes
- Rowing Time: 15 minutes
    - For this workout you are going to get off the rower as well to help prevent injuries and work the other muscles!
    - Row for 5:00, 3 times. In between each 5-minute piece, you will get off the rower and do:
        - 1:00 plank
        - 15 push-ups

# BEGINNER'S GUIDE TO ROWING

- 20 squats
  - So row 5:00, get off and do the three exercises above, row another 5:00, get off and do exercises, row 5:00, get off and do exercises.
- Afterwards, record:
  - Total meters rowed after each?

  - How did it feel?

  - What SPM did you settle at for each?

## Week 4
**Workout 1:**
Overview:
- Total Time: Roughly 15 minutes.
- Rowing Time: Roughly 15 minutes.
  - Row for 2 minutes at 20 SPM, nice and gentle.
  - Row another 2 minutes at whatever SPM you would like, but nice and gentle.
  - Reset your monitor screen so it's easy to follow along.
  - Row at a SPM of 16, for 1 minute. Then for the next minute, row at a SPM of 17. Then the next minute, row at a SPM of 18. Keep increasing until you get to a SPM of 22, which should take you to the 7-minute mark.
  - Then switch to increasing your stroke rate by 1, every 30 seconds instead of every minute, until you get to a final stroke rate of 30 SPM for 30 seconds.
  - Cool down.
- Afterwards, record:
  - How did it feel? Tired? Out of breath? Need a break?

  - Total time and meters rowed?

  - What was your average split time?

**Workout 2:**

BEGINNER'S GUIDE TO ROWING

Overview:
- Total Time: Roughly 30 minutes
- Rowing Time: Under 30 minutes
    - Row 3000 meters
    - Find a pace that is comfortable. Focus on your breathing. Focus on form.
- Afterwards, record:
    - Average Pace?
    - How long did it take?
    - Average SPM that was comfortable?
    - How did it feel? Need breaks? Out of breath?

**Workout 3:**

Overview:
- Total Time: Roughly 15 minutes
- Rowing Time: Roughly 15 minutes
    - Row 100 meters, 20 times, without any breaks if you can. Try to keep the SPM below 24 for the entire workout!
    - So...
        - Row 100 meters hard (really pushing through your legs, but not speeding up on the SPM).
        - Then row 100 meters, nice and easy (so it's like a break, but you are still moving).
        - Then repeat 100 meters hard, 100 meters easy, on and off until 20 times, which will be 2000 meters.
- Afterwards, record:
    - Total time it took to row?
    - Average SPM you settled at?
    - How did it feel?

## Chapter 11: FREQUENTLY ASKED QUESTIONS

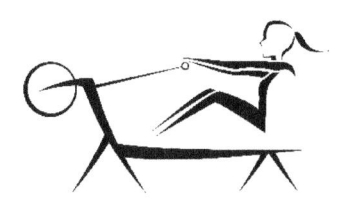

*There is no such thing as a dumb question.*
                                           - Carl Sagan

# Chapter 11: Frequently Asked Questions!

I get a lot of questions about rowing and I wanted to share some of the most frequently asked questions and my thoughts with you here. If you have questions of your own, please feel free to reach out in the Keep Rowing Longer! Facebook group.

## What shoes should I wear?

This is a really common question in athletes and it also varies from person to person, however I will give a brief overview of some pros and cons of certain types of shoes in regards to rowing on the indoor rowing machine. There are so many different types of shoes these days that I won't be able to cover them all, but I will cover the basics.

*Weightlifting Shoes*

Most people don't use weightlifting shoes when rowing, however I am starting with these shoes for a reason. Weightlifting shoes have a raised heel, which is basically a heel lift. This heel lift makes it so that when you are squatting, if you have decreased ankle mobility, it is easier to squat lower. The catch position in rowing puts you in a similar position to that of a squat. So if you have decreased ankle mobility, you might think that having something with a heel lift would be beneficial. While this is the case, you are better off playing around with the footplate positioning, which is discussed in Chapter 5.

The other pro to weightlifting shoes is that they have a hard sole, which in terms of weightlifting allows less force and energy to be lost through the cushion in your shoe. Rowing is similar, where you want to have as much force production through your feet as you can, so rowing with a hard sole could be helpful.

However, the pro of a stiff, hard-soled weightlifting shoe is also the negative in regards to these shoes. This stiffness doesn't allow you to go up on your toes at all, so you will lose movement, as you won't be able to get as far up at the catch position. However, for some people it is helpful to learn to row with your entire foot remaining on the footplate, but in the long run, you will usually have your heels come up and that is very difficult in a stiff-soled shoe.

*Running Sneakers*

Running shoes are soft, comfy, and flexible. Because of this, they seem like the perfect shoe. They don't have the stiffness issue that weightlifting shoes have, however, because there is usually so much cushion in the sole of the shoe, you will inevitably lose a little bit of force production to the sole of the shoe when rowing. However, this loss in force is so small that the average rower won't notice a difference and it won't make a big change. However if you are training for something, you might want to keep this in mind.

*Barefoot (no shoes)*

Many people are starting to run and workout barefoot these days. While that is great, and it solves the soft cushion issue with rowing, it doesn't feel that great on your heel or Achilles and some people end up with sores or blisters on the back of their heel. This is because the heel strap to help keep your foot on the footplate rubs continuously on your heel. Some people do put some type of foam cushion there and some people just row anyway. If it doesn't bother your heel, then fantastic, but if it does, I would recommend finding a shoe to help. Even wearing socks will often still result in a sore on the heel.

*Metcons*

Metcons are really common in the CrossFit world. They give you a harder sole, but also provide some support to your foot and cushioning around the Achilles area. I think these are great for rowing because it's a nice mix in the middle for people. Your ankle isn't likely to get roughed up, and you have improved force production without losing force to the cushion.

Ultimately choosing the right shoe is going to vary from person to person and I recommend finding a shoe that is comfortable for you. For instance, I have had three left ankle surgeries and have a scar on the back of my heel along the Achilles. If I row barefoot or without cushion on the back of my heel, I won't be rowing very long as it will be uncomfortable. I also need a lot of cushion for repetitive motions where I am pushing through my feet, so I use running sneakers. Find what is comfortable and works for you and your body.

## I walk duck-footed - what should I do?

I actually love helping people with this. This is the perfect example of people needing to adjust the rowing machine for them, which is what I talk about in this book.

Earlier in this book I talked about adapting the machine and how there are certain things you can change and certain things you can't. If you walk with your feet pointed outwards, and then you force your feet to be pointed forward when they are on the foot stretcher, it's like forcing yourself to walk with your feet pointed forward. Have you tried to do that, because a lot of my clients have, and they say it's pretty difficult.

So if it's hard to keep your toes pointed forward walking, you should not do it rowing. You might be wondering, "What do I do then?" Great question!

The key is the straps on the footplate. First, loosen the straps, like a lot! Then put your feet in, but instead of forcing your feet to point forward, let them fall out to the angle that is comfortable for you. Then tighten the straps, but only so much that your feet aren't forced to move into the position we are trying to avoid. So now when you row, your toes should be pointed out a bit more, as if you are in a position that you would walk. Tada! Now try rowing. Does it feel better?

The downside to forcing your feet to point forward is that you might be leading yourself to the possibility of injuries from forcing your legs to be in a position over and over again that it doesn't want to be in and the reason will vary from person to person. For some, it's because your hip joint is angled a little differently, for some it's a foot issue, etc. There are lots of reasons you might walk duck-footed, but by changing the position of your feet, you are decreasing the likelihood of an overuse injury in your feet, ankles, shins, knees, hips, and back.

## I get tailbone rashes - what do I do?

Tailbone rashes often happen for a couple of reasons. The first is that you might not be sitting on your sit bones, so instead your pelvis is tilted and you are more on your tailbone. So when you go back and forth through the rowing stroke, you are causing a rubbing and shearing force on your tailbone, which causes friction and leads to sores. So first thing, check out the pelvis section in Chapter 5 and make sure you have adjusted your buttocks into a good position.

The second reason might be because of your clothing. If you have clothing that is rubbing and causing friction, you might want to try something tight like spandex, which will help reduce any friction from your clothes.

The last reason you might have rashes on your buttocks is because you have a bony buttocks. Add some muscle from strength training and that might help. But ideally you shouldn't be getting rashes, it should just be a "sore bum" and it should improve as you row more. It is similar to cycling. When cycling, the seat hurts for a while, but then your body adapts to the seat and it doesn't hurt as much. The same goes for the rowing seat. Give it time and your buttocks will start to adapt.

**I have a belly or am pregnant - what should I do?**

So do I! I have a belly. I'm not pregnant. But if this is you, the key is to adapt the rowing stroke to better fit your body type. Check out Chapter 5 and 6 for a little info on how to adapt and adjust the machine. However, let me touch on this subject a little more here.

If you have a belly, you might want to bring your legs out to the side when you are at the catch, so that you can get more range of motion from the stroke. I don't recommend this. Instead, when you get to the catch, stop before your legs start to come out. What this means is that your stroke will be a little shorter, but that is okay. Just go as far forward as you can without changing your form from your back or your legs. This might even make it so your heels don't come up, which is fine. You can also try moving the foot plate a notch or two downward, and that might help you get in a more comfortable position as well. But try your best to keep the regular positioning; just don't go as far forward at the catch.

If you are pregnant, it's the same thing, except let your knees come out a little, but not so much that your knees are all the way at your shoulders. When you are pregnant, your ligaments actually become a little more lax, and this leads to increased flexibility, but also sometimes leads to pain. So you

## I get back pain - is this normal?

Unfortunately, back pain with rowing is really common. However, it doesn't need to be! Remember: focus on form! The primary reason that people get back pain with rowing is because of form errors. Leaning too far back, rounding the back at the catch, or starting the rowing stroke with their shoulders moving back instead of really pushing with the legs first.[1]

If this is the case, please feel free to reach out in the Facebook group or message me and I would be happy to help, but back pain does not need to be a part of rowing. In fact, rowing should help strengthen the core and back, resulting in decreased back pain. So if you have back pain, please look at your form, record yourself, and figure out where your form might be going a little haywire.

## I had back surgery - can I row?

First off, I do recommend checking in with your surgeon and having a conversation. Just like the question before this, many people, doctors included, say don't row after back surgery. However, I don't believe this is universally true. There have been studies showing that activity is beneficial in helping to reduce fear avoidance behaviors and that movement helps reduce chronic back pain symptoms.[23, 24] Saying someone can't or shouldn't do something may be appropriate medical advice, but it can also instill fear and delay recovery. It's your body, your recovery, so don't be afraid to discuss alternatives and ask your surgeon for his or her reasoning or for more information. Definitely check with your surgeon, but some also may not fully understand rowing themselves, so have the discussion with them if rowing is something that you want to try or want to return to.

Rowing is similar to squatting, which you do everyday when going up and down from a chair. It is also similar to a deadlift, which has been shown to decrease back pain when loaded and done correctly.[25] So if rowing is a mix of those two movements, then why should you be scared of them? You also deadlift and squat when you pick a pencil or box up from the ground. Rowing is great at helping with back strength, so as long as you focus on form. As I mentioned in the previous question, just start slow, focus on form, and you will get there.[1] That being said, I wouldn't recommend starting by rowing 5,000 meters everyday, or a half marathon or more, but slowly ease in, focus on form, and feel free to reach out if you want help in this regard.

## I get blisters - should I wear gloves or use chalk to help keep the handle from slipping?

Sorry, but unfortunately blisters are part of rowing. However, first, you want to figure out where your blisters are. And you might be thinking, "on my hands, duh." That's great, but where on your hands?

A common cause of blisters from indoor rowing is from gripping the handle a little too hard, which is discussed more in depth in Chapter 5. If your blisters are in the middle of your hand, over-gripping is likely the culprit. If your blisters are a little closer to your fingers, or on your fingers, then it might just be your delicate hands getting used to rowing. Pace yourself, those blisters will transform into a badge of honor!

When it comes to gloves and chalk, I don't recommend it. The gloves are a little less of an issue on the indoor rowing machine than they are on the water, but ultimately, you might end up over-gripping without noticing. Having your hands be gloveless will allow you to critique your form and work on things more than letting a glove "mask" the issue.

Similar to gloves, I don't recommend chalk because it will actually increase the friction in the area and can make blisters worse. However, the main reason I don't like chalk is because it leaves residue on the handle and if you have a machine that you share with others, you are forcing other people to use chalk, when that might not be ideal for their hands. If you have your own machine, and chalk works, then go for it! But if you share machines, please keep this in mind.

## I want to buy a rower – do you have any recommendations?

I get this question a lot and I will answer this to the best of my abilities here. First off, there are four different types of rowing machines and they are classified based on the type of resistance they use: magnetic, air, hydraulic, or water.[26] Different people tend to prefer one over the other, or are looking for a bargain and choose one based on that. In my opinion, the best way to choose a rower is to try a few out. Go to a local fitness studio or gym equipment store and try the rowers that they have. Some people love the sound of the whoosh whoosh that the water-based rowers make. Some people like the quietness of some of the magnetic machines. It really is about your personal preference. I do talk about the WaterRower and Concept2 in this book because they are the most common ones, but I will talk about them more here too. With that in mind, let me give you a brief overview of the different types of resistance.

*Magnetic Resistance*

These are usually the quietest machines, so if that is important to you, you might want to look at these types of rowers. These machines usually give you a smooth rowing feeling as well. They use magnets and a spinning flywheel to change the resistance you feel on the machine. The biggest disadvantage to these machines is that they don't really simulate water rowing as much, but if you just want a good workout, go for it. As long as your criteria are met, then yay! I talk more about the criteria later in this section.[26]

*Air Resistance*

Air resistance is the most popular type of rowing machine. The resistance is based on airflow through a flywheel, so as you pull, the flywheel spins. The more power you put into your stroke, the faster the flywheel spins. These machines also have a form of damper setting, mentioned earlier in this book. Air resistance machines are good at replicating rowing on the water, the resistance adjusts with your rowing, it's smooth, and it usually needs less maintenance. The downside is that these machines are usually a little louder than other options.[26] The Concept2 is an example of this type of machine and is considered the "gold standard" with rowing machines.

The Concept2 is the most common machine used in CrossFit boxes, Row House, and erg rooms for people who do the sport of crew. The way this machine feels is pretty similar to being on the water and the numbers correlate very well to numbers that people would get when rowing on the water. So people competing often use this machine. Concept2 also has an online database to compare times with other people and competitions throughout the year as well. Most of the apps that are created for the indoor rowing machine are compatible with the Concept2. However, this machine is a little more expensive, with a current price tag of roughly USD $900.[27] People will search for these machines to go on sale, and they get purchased fairly quickly, however this machine holds its value fairly well and can have multiple millions of meters on it and still work great. Even though this machine feels like being on the water, it uses air resistance, not water.

## BEGINNER'S GUIDE TO ROWING

*Hydraulic Resistance*

These rowing machines are usually at a lower price point and are often quiet as well. These machines will still give you a good workout, but they aren't very comfortable or as smooth as the other options. The hydraulic rowing mechanism uses pistons that are attached to the handles, and you pull against the air or fluid in the cylinder, and levels or clamps change the resistance. A downside is that the resistance will not stay consistent, as the oil heats up, the resistance will change. These rowing machines often have two handles as well, which can be nice if you want that type of movement. Another thing to keep in mind is that these machines often need more maintenance.[26]

*Water Resistance*

Water rowers use paddles in the water as their form of resistance. There is water in a tank, and when you pull on the handle, the paddles move the water. The mass of the water moving creates a drag and therefore creates resistance. Similar to air resistance machines, the more power you put, the more the water moves. These machines are usually quieter than an air-based machine, are nice and smooth, and sound nice. There is also little maintenance needed with these machines.

The WaterRower is an example of this type of machine. There are water rowers that are not this brand, but the brand WaterRower is the next most common water based rowing machine that people get, and is roughly the same price as a Concept2, currently at USD $895.[28] People love the sound this machine makes, as it makes you feel like you are on the water. If you are going to get this machine, there are some things you might want to consider. First, the footplate is actually a little narrower than it is on some other machines. So, if you have wider hips or shoulders, this is something to consider. I mentioned it earlier in the book, but this position can cause you to compensate a little if you are not careful. There are some footplate extenders you can get that are a little wider, but it is an extra cost, but definitely something to consider if you need it. Second, the seat is a little higher, so it changes the angles at your ankles, knees, and hips. Not bad, just different. And lastly, the screen is down low on many models, so if you look at the numbers a lot, it might take a toll on your neck. But the WaterRower comes in steel or wood, looks nice, and sounds cool.[28] There are also some apps that work with this machine, so keep that in mind too. Not as many as with the Concept2, but still more than with off brand rowers.

    Now let's cover the "off" brand rowers. Pretty much any other brand is an "off" brand rower, such as: Lifestyle, NordicTrack, Sunny Health & Fitness, Stamina, etc. There really are so many that I won't list them all. Each is a little different, but knowing the resistance differences might help point you in the right direction. Some of the key things to pay attention to are: how does it feel, do the numbers tell you the info you want, is it in the price range you want, and does it have all the features you want? For example, if you want to hook up to a program like ErgRow that monitors your meters, not all machines will do that. Same with hooking up a heart rate monitor, they won't all do that either. If a machine doesn't tell you the split or pace like mentioned earlier in this book, I personally wouldn't buy it, as it won't give you numbers that are helpful in setting goals and seeing improvements.

    Regardless of the machine, every one varies in how it feels, so I recommend trying them out if you can. If you are going to look for a rowing machine on sale, Facebook Marketplace, Craigslist, indoor rowing competitions, and local Facebook CrossFit groups are great for searching. Depending on the machine, there are different things to look for. The basics include: does the screen turn on and work? Does the seat slide smoothly? Is it broken or chipped at all? Have they been keeping up with maintenance?

I hope that helps and feel free to reach out if you have questions!

# BEGINNER'S GUIDE TO ROWING

## Want help or have questions?

If you are more of a visual person, or you simply want personal assistance, one-on-one guidance or accountability, we offer rowing consults and a rowing program to improve your stamina that complements what you've learned in this book. Additionally, you can find some videos on my YouTube channel.

There is also a free Facebook group called, *Keep Rowing Longer!*, where you can ask your questions and get guidance. You can access all of this at my website (link below).

I really hope you enjoyed this book and found it beneficial. Please leave a review to let me know how I can improve and how to help others find this book.

**Links:**

Website: www.rowingdoc.com

Facebook group:
https://www.facebook.com/groups/rowinglonger/

YouTube Channel:
https://www.youtube.com/channel/UCb0crIZU9cLyGCxcJPYqcLA

# Products

## Rowing Consults

We offer one-on-one rowing consults, which can also be with injury prevention assistance. This can be done via video such as skype/facetime and is a great way to help you solidify your form while you continue to improve and also help avoid injury by getting another person's perspective from the beginning.

## Forever Rowing

Forever Rowing is the course that goes along with this book and is designed to help you row 30+ minutes without being out of breath. It is a 5-week program with four weeks' worth of workouts, with five workouts per week; plus access to a private Facebook group with extra guidance from me. If you are interested in this program and would like a 25% discount, email me at: Amanda@rowingdoc.com

## Rowing for PTs and Coaches

This is our program designed for Physical Therapists and coaches to help you to help your clients avoid injury and includes training to help you spot form errors so you can better help your clients stay pain-free on the rower.

## Resilient Rower

This is a flexibility and mobility program designed for rowers to help you stay active and mobile on and off the rowing machine. Taking care of our bodies takes time, and this helps you target the areas that rowers need to work on the most to help you get a great routine without wasting your time. If you have injuries, it will help you focus on an area as well.

# BEGINNER'S GUIDE TO ROWING

BEGINNER'S GUIDE TO ROWING

This book was written with the assistance of Jeremy Sutton of Healthy Books, LLC.

Jeremy is a physical therapist. He is the creator of Healthcare Self-Publishing Academy where he teaches healthcare providers how to become the seen authority in their profession and their region. Join the free Facebook group Healthcare Self-Publishing Academy to learn how to get your book written and published. You can set up a discovery call on his website to learn how you can get your book done in 90 days.

*Telling Your Story Starts Here*

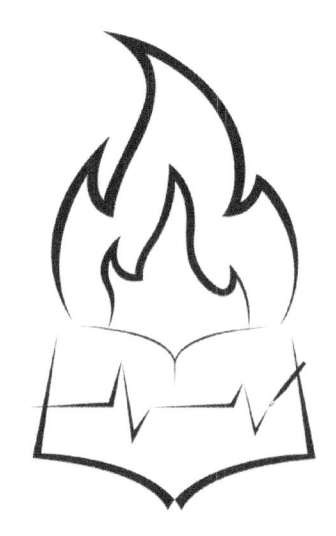

HEALTHCARE SELF PUBLISHING ACADEMY

WWW.HEALTHYBOOKS.NET

WWW.FACEBOOK.COM/SELFPUBLISHINGACADEMY

# BEGINNER'S GUIDE TO ROWING

## References

1. Hosea TM, Hannafin JA. Rowing Injuries. *Sports Health: A Multidisciplinary Approach.* 2012;4(3):236-245. Doi:10.1177/1941738112442484
2. Danny. History of the Rowing Machine. Rowing & Fitness website. https://www.rowing-machine-review.com/history-of-the-rowing-machine/. Published December 26, 2018. Accessed October 10, 2020.
3. Low Impact Testimonials. Concept2 website. https://www.concept2.com/indoor-rowers/testimonials/category/low-impact. Accessed December 10, 2020.
4. Feito Y, Burrows EK, Tabb LP. A 4-Year Analysis of the Incidence of Injuries Among CrossFit-Trained Participants. Orthopaedic journal of sports medicine. https://www.ncbi.nlm.nih.gov/pmc/articles/PMC6201188/. Published October 24, 2018. Accessed January 20, 2020.
5. Young, MD C. 7 Common Indoor Cycling Injuries. Medscape website. https://reference.medscape.com/features/slideshow/indoor-cycling-injuries. Accessed January 20, 2020.
6. Rowing Basics. Princeton National Rowing Association website. https://www.rowpnra.org/pnra/rowing-basics/. Accessed January 22, 2020.
7. Cheri. Using the Force Curve. Concept2. https://www.concept2.com/indoor-rowers/training/tips-and-general-info/using-the-force-curve. Published July 24, 2019. Accessed January 20, 2020.
8. How to Use Your PM4. Concept2 website. https://www.concept2.com/service/monitors/pm4/how-to-use/using-monitor-display-options. Accessed December 20, 2020.
9. Workout Types. HowToRow website. https://www.howtorow.com/workouts/. Accessed January 20, 2020.

10. Cheri. Damper Setting 101. Concept2 website. https://www.concept2.com/indoor-rowers/training/tips-and-general-info/damper-setting-101. Published July 24, 2019. Accessed January 24, 2020.
11. Huang M, Hajizadeh K, Gibson I, Lee T. Analysis of compressive load on intervertebral joint in standing and sitting postures. *Technology and Healthcare.* 2016;24(2):215-223. doi:10.3233/THC-151100.
12. Cheri. Technique Videos. Concept2 website. https://www.concept2.com/indoor-rowers/training/technique-videos. Published August 2, 2019. Accessed January 20, 2020.
13. Meredith. Rowing is a Leg Sport. Concept2 website. https://www.concept2.com/news/rowing-leg-sport-0. Published June 4, 2018. Accessed December 26, 2020.
14. Low Impact Exercises For Shin Splints. Shin Splints Clinic website. http://www.shinsplintsclinic.com/low-impact-exercises-for-shin-splints/. Published April 9, 2017. Accessed January 24, 2020.
15. Patel H, Alkhawam H, Madanieh R, Shah N, Kosmas CE, Vittorio TJ. Aerobic vs anaerobic exercise training effects on the cardiovascular system. World Journal of Cardiology. 2017;9(2):134-138. doi:10.4330/wjc.v9.i2.134.
16. Foster C, Farland CV, Guidotti F, et al. The Effects of High Intensity Interval Training vs Steady State Training on Aerobic and Anaerobic Capacity. Journal of Sports Science & Medicine. 2015;14(4):747-755.
17. High-Intensity Interval Training: Meaning of High-Intensity Interval Training by Lexico. Lexico Dictionaries | English website. https://www.lexico.com/definition/high-intensity_interval_training. Accessed January 24, 2020.
18. Tabata: Meaning of Tabata by Lexico. Lexico Dictionaries | English website. https://www.lexico.com/definition/tabata. Accessed January 24, 2020.

19. Judy. 7 Reasons to Include Intervals in your Workouts. Concept2 website. https://www.concept2.com/news/7-reasons-to-include-intervals-your-workouts. Published January 16, 2020. Accessed January 24, 2020.
20. Linoby A, Zaki MSM, Baki H, et al. The Effects of High-Intensity Interval Training and Continuous Training on Weight Loss and Body Composition in Overweight Females. SpringerLink. https://link.springer.com/chapter/10.1007/978-981-287-107-7_42. Published January 1, 1970. Accessed January 24, 2020.
21. De Feo P. Is high-intensity exercise better than moderate-intensity exercise for weight loss? Nutrition, Metabolism & Cardiovascular Diseases. 2013;23(11):1037-1042. doi:10.1016/j.numecd.2013.06.002.
22. Cheri. Breathing Techniques. Concept2 website. https://www. concept2.com/indoor-rowers/training/tips-and-general-info/breathing-techniques. Published July 24, 2019. Accessed January 20, 2020.
23. Hazard RG. Failed Back Surgery Syndrome: Surgical and Nonsurgical Approaches. *Clinical Orthopaedics and Related Research*. 2006;443:228-232. doi:10.1097/01.blo.0000200230.46071.3d.
24. Aasa B, Berglund L, Michaelson P, Aasa U. Individualized low-load motor control exercises and education versus a high-load lifting exercise and education to improve activity, pain intensity, and physical performance in patients with low back pain: a randomized controlled trial. *Journal of Orthopaedic and Sports Physical Therapy*. 2015;45(2):77-85. doi:10.2519/jospt.2015.5021.
25. Reikerås O, Storheim K, Holm I, Friis A, Brox JI. Disability, Pain, Psychological Factors And Physical Performance In Healthy Controls, Patients With Sub-Acute And Chronic Low Back Pain: A Case-Control

Study. *Journal of Rehabilitation Medicine.* 2005;37(2):95-99. doi:10.1080/16501970410017738.
26. Rowing Machine Resistance Types. Home Rowing Machine Reviews 2020 website. https://www.rowingmachine-guide.com/types.html. Accessed February 6, 2020.
27. Model D Indoor Rower. Concept2 website. Accessed February 6, 2020.
28. Shop. View All WaterRower Models and Prices website. https://www.waterrower.com/us/shop.html. Accessed February 6, 2020.

Printed in Great Britain
by Amazon